Apple Cider Vinegar for Health and Wellness

The Simple Remedy that Helps You Lose Weight, Clear Your Skin, and Boost Your Immune System

Kathryn Young

Special Bonus

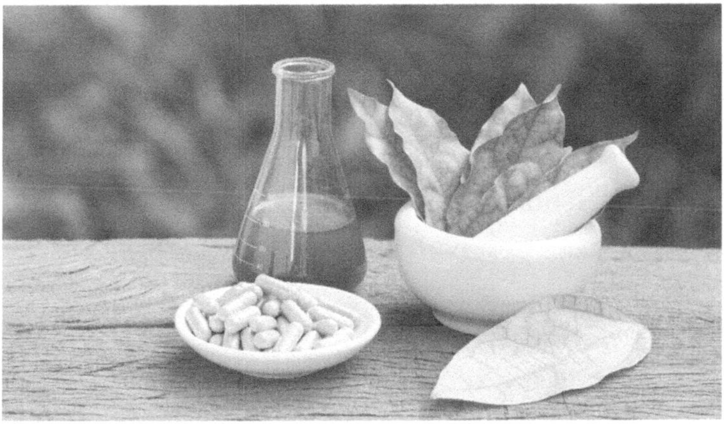

Get the Bonus Report that includes:

- ❑ Weight loss supplement buying guide
- ❑ Why **MOST** diets fail
- ❑ Alternative medicine tricks that worked for me

Get it now, visit the link:

bit.ly/healthybonus

Table of Contents

Introduction

"I adopted a healthier diet; I take at least a tablespoon of apple cider vinegar a day. It's an old wives' tale, but it really is one of the best things you can put in your mouth."

— Mellisa Etheridge

It is incredible how a simple change in personal choices can significantly change life altogether. We have heard about such changes in stories and inspirational videos quite a lot, but we are in the habit of taking most of these with a pinch of salt.

I was exactly in the same boat as you. I hardly believed anything I read and skipped past quite a few of these so-called life-altering methods. It was only recently that I kept on hearing about this 'new thing' that apparently did work. I kept hearing people praise how pleasing the results were and how many of them were actually able to lose weight and look better than ever before. Needless to say, it got me a little curious, and hence I started looking into the world of apple cider vinegar (ACV).

If I were to define the results in just one sentence, it would sound something like this: *"You have to try it to believe it!"*

However, instead of just advertising ACV and how incredible it is, I decided to share something a little more meaningful. *Apple Cider Vinegar for Health and Wellness*, therefore, is the result.

Unlike any other diet you may have heard of, this one is not aimed at starving you to near-death, nor is it seeking to make you feel like you are being punished for putting on a few pounds. It is downright the most straightforward way of changing your life without all that hassle and stress.

Through this book, I intend to unveil the original beauty that lies within the use of ACV and explain just why everyone is so eager to talk about it. Together, we will go through various examples, backed by scientific facts and data, and eventually see if ACV indeed lives up to its reputation. After all, in matters that impact our lives, we must only choose the best there is.

The science here is not just about the chemicals involved and how they work to bring out the most exceptional results, but in something that is often overlooked. There are things we all must know and abide by to ensure we only end up reaping the benefits and not the harm that it can cause. I have found some cases where people, fascinated by the quick results, decided to up the dose without prior consultation or thought. Get the balance wrong, and you start facing some backlashes. That is where this book comes in, to help you identify what you need to do and how much must be done to see the results.

I will also share some interesting statistics, facts, and references that will show just how effective ACV really is and why we need it in our lives. And that brings us to the burning question — why should you read this book over all the others?

What Does This Book Offer?

Before writing this book, I had done my fair share of research and taken into account my personal experiences and those of my close acquaintances to learn just how effective ACV is. Through this book, I aim to share all the in-depth knowledge about the ACV science, the facts, the advantages, the benefits, as well as things you should keep an eye out for.

Many books go to great lengths to praise specific methods, but they never provide complete information. I have seen blog entries, hundreds of them, and most talk only about the positive aspects. I genuinely believe that to fully explore the science behind ACV, one should also discover the side less talked about.

By providing comprehensive information, along with some tasty recipes and delightful trivia facts, you should soon be in a comfortable position to decide whether ACV is for you or not.

For those seeking ways to shed off weight, let me assure you that apple cider vinegar is one incredible find. Whoever came up with this discovery, I wish to let them know they did the world a massive favor.

We will talk in detail regarding the numerous advantages and benefits of ACV. We will also look into some crucial and highly recommended lifestyle choices, such as holistic living. We will dive into the world of acne and find out just how ACV helps us with acne problems. If you are someone who suffers from heart-related issues and fluctuating blood sugar levels, keep reading, as you would certainly be surprised to know just how beneficial ACV can be for you.

With so much to offer, it's hard to resist the temptation of taking a peek into the world of apple cider vinegar. Once you start reading, it is quite hard to resist trying it out yourself. If you feel such an urge at any point, you are more than welcome to begin your transformational journey. It does not take a rocket scientist to figure out that this method is indeed worth the hype as it would be evidently clear in a matter of weeks.

Oh, I almost forgot! Try to take notes where and when possible. You might, at times, be in a place where you may not be carrying your copy of the book. A quick and handy notepad or notes app on your phone should provide you with all you need to carry on without problems.

Furthermore, the recipes provided within this book are just a sample. They are there to serve as a great starting point for you, just so that you can have a taste of what to expect. There are well over thousands of recipes, tips, and tricks, some of which are covered within this book. Browse the internet for any additional recipes or tips you wish to look for.

Finally, I have done my best to ensure that I do not end up using terminologies that are far too vague or difficult for the general audience to understand. I have taken every effort to use simple terms and, where used, I have tried to explain things so that they are as easy to understand as possible. If you still feel stuck, be sure to check with our good friend, Google (or any other search engine of your choice).

About the Author

My name is Kathryn Young. I am a fitness blogger by passion and a personal trainer. Ever since I can remember, I have always felt my passion for health deeply rooted, and it is because of this that I find pleasure in getting to know and learn all about how to optimize health to boost our body's performance.

This passion of mine led me to pursue nutrition, and soon enough, I became a registered dietitian. While things were moving in the direction I had wanted, I soon felt as if something was off. With a bit of in-depth research and additional knowledge, I learned how even though the physical aspect of fitness remained important, a well-balanced consumption of food and drink was simply beyond compare.

I continued digging deep and went through numerous scientific studies. These studies primarily focused on the body's natural ability to produce energy and perform tasks. That search continued on and soon converted into a personal mission; a mission where I wanted to gather as much information as I could, and then use that sea of information to help others learn more about optimizing their health for improved physical performance.

Apple Cider Vinegar for Health and Wellness is the fruit of my hard work and labor. It is the summarized result of all that I have learned and acquired throughout the years. Whether it delivers on that front or not is up to you to decide. With that said, let us leave my introduction aside and get straight to business. Let us start our journey towards the goal that brought you here in the first place, the world of apple cider vinegar!

Chapter 1:

Holistic Living 101

Before we actually begin with the entire apple cider vinegar concept, there are a few things we should get to know better. Consider these as prerequisites; they significantly help in achieving the desired results faster and with more success.

Living life is only a distant dream if you have poor health. While many think a person's health has more to do with the way they look, the finer details require a little introduction.

Health is quite a broad term. It covers so many aspects, all combined and working together to produce a result that is either good or bad. Take an example of two people, Mr. A and Mr. B.

Both are 33 years old, single, and have a good source of income. Mr. A is a person who has some extra pounds, while Mr. B is rather skinny. Who do you think is leading a healthier life here?

There would be some who say Mr. A, while others may say that Mr. B is leading a better life. Your physical health or shape is only a part of a bigger story here. There is a possibility both might be leading a healthy life, and equally another side that might prove both are leading unhealthy lifestyles.

A healthy person is one who has a good physical, emotional, and mental state. Added to that, holistic living brings your soul into the mix as well. Confused? Let's look a little deeper to further understand what I am on about.

Holistic living simply means living as a whole person. Instead of just focusing on reducing or gaining weight, holistic living promotes everyone to pay more attention to the entire human being: mind, body, and soul. Take one away, and you can never truly lead a happy, stress-free, and successful life.

In some regions of the world, holistic living has been misinterpreted as a way of living where you devote your life to strengthening your soul while giving up on all the worldly charms and pleasures. Yes, this holistic approach does teach you how to be happy from the inside, but it never limits you to that alone.

Holistic living is a concept that looks upon a person as a whole. From petty things such as eating something you like to something as significant as moving to a different city, everything is looked upon through various angles to figure out which works the best for the person as a whole. This means that if something pleases your body, your mind, and your soul, it is something certainly worth the effort. Anything else that upsets the balance, it is best to walk away from.

The rather difficult journey takes quite some time before you truly start feeling the results. Eventually, you will find that holistic ways encourage you to be more confident, be more in control of your life than you thought possible, and be able to do things you never dreamt of doing before.

A holistic way of living pushes one to look at every factor that can end up affecting us as complex beings. This then covers pretty much everything you can think of, such as what you might eat, how you might sleep, whom you may meet, your relationships, your way of thinking, and how you manage your stress. If I was to define the core idea of the entire holistic living concept in one sentence, it would be this: *Establish a connection between your mind and body to optimize health.*

Achieving that, however, is no ordinary task but also not as difficult as people might think. All it takes is a bit of dedication, some basic knowledge about a few things, and determination. Just as all good things take time and effort, the holistic lifestyle requires consistency and perseverance. Stating that the results are worth it is an understatement, and that is saying something.

So what exactly are the advantages of leading a holistic lifestyle? Why are quite a lot of people so eager to publicize this way of living, and is it actually any different? These are some of the questions I get asked by so many people I know. While holistic living comes with quite a few advantages, some stand out above others, such as:

- An improved overall health
- A well-balanced life
- A more profound connection with nature and soul
- Better diet intake
- Pain relief through various exercises

I have barely scratched the surface of the never-ending advantages the holistic lifestyle has for everyone. Since our prime focus within this book is on ACV, adding holistic living can bring some of the finest results you can expect in life. And, with that said, it is time for us to crack the code to the holistic lifestyle and see how one can begin leading such a life that seems to hold so many promising benefits. I will walk you through some significant components involved in the holistic habits and cover some essential details to ensure you know exactly where to begin and how to proceed from here on out.

The Major Components Behind Health and Wellness

While I can put forward quite an extensive list of said components which work together to bring the results we all desire out of the holistic lifestyle, it would be overwhelming and perhaps a little too advanced for now. For us to begin our journey, we first need to identify these significant components which serve as the foundation of the entire 'living as a whole' theory.

All of these do not require you to have special skills or knowledge to experience them yourself. All you need is determination and a will that keeps you moving forward.

Exercise

When anyone talks about health and wellbeing, the first thing that naturally hits our head is exercise. It goes without saying that exercising regularly holds far more advantages than one can count. It helps you remain calm and composed. It helps to alleviate any stress that you might be suffering from. It is a perfect way to change your mood and feel alive again.

Exercise is not only meant for people who are either looking to reduce their weight or gain some muscle, but it's meant for every individual, regardless of their body weight and type. As we progress ahead, you will come to learn just how many issues can be resolved through healthy exercise routines.

Whether you are male or female, looking good and feeling good about yourself is your birthright. It is unfortunate that with time, we tend to overlook the needs of our bodies and are more focused on meeting the needs to satisfy our minds.

Besides, exercises greatly help in reducing the chances of suffering from various medical ailments as well. If you are someone who suffers from cardiac issues or has active type 2 diabetes, exercise is the first step to take. According to reports (Semeco, 2017), some prominent benefits of exercising on a daily basis include:

- Reduced risk of heart attack
- Better weight management
- Lower blood pressure
- Lower blood cholesterol levels
- Lower risk of some cancer types
- Strengthens bones and muscles, hence reducing the risk of osteoporosis
- Better recovery
- Better sleep
- Makes one feel more relaxed

These are quite a handful of benefits, all of which are too tempting for anyone suffering from any of these conditions. I know you might be thinking that you can never find the time to work out regularly. I was in the same boat as you, but then I managed my time to ensure I could squeeze out an hour every other day.

Eventually, I was able to manage an hour every day and started seeing the results myself. The results were fascinating, to say the least. I felt much better about myself. I was more confident wherever I went because I knew I would look better than I did before I worked out. It automatically had an impact on the people around me as they started noticing these small changes. I was genuinely surprised to see just how much exercising regularly can help a person.

Apart from the above, regular exercises allow you to have a healthy state of mind. Your body is already taking in its share of the goodness and, simultaneously, so is your mind.

There have been a few studies on how exactly exercise helps the human mind, and almost all of them concluded that exercise helps in fighting depression, a common plague found in every other person you meet.

Depression is real and can lead to devastating consequences if not treated accordingly. Exercise is perhaps the greatest way to help you feel better and come out of this dreadful state. It's one of the best ways to take your mind off the worries and daily stress we all experience. If you are someone who thinks of exercising regularly but procrastinates a bit, it is time to put your foot down and go for it. The more you delay, the more time you lose, and that is something none of us can afford.

Sleep

This is something most of us just love to do. Some may not know this, but as tempting as a peaceful sleep is, it is one of the hardest things to get. We do sleep, but sleeping at the wrong time, in the wrong circumstances, and with the wrong thoughts before bed can significantly affect how our body utilizes our sleep. Rest is far more than just slumber on a comfortable bed. This is the time when our body actually recovers all the energy it needs to handle the next day. However, sleep a little more than usual, and you wake up with a few sore muscles.

Sleep is perhaps the most essential part of our daily life. Without it, we would never regain our energy, and we would end up losing focus. Needless to say, if you had little sleep, you would wake up feeling irritated by almost everything around you. Even the best morning person will feel precisely the same. Striking a balance, therefore, is vital to make the most of our sleep.

There are a few things we all need to ensure if we genuinely wish to experience a peaceful slumber, and they are:

- **Sleeping at natural times** - Sleeping during or in the middle of the day is not a good option for our body.

- **Keeping all the distractions away** - If you wish to allow your body to heal, recover, and, at the same time, enjoy sleep itself, be sure to keep all distractions away.

- **Sleep six to eight hours at most** - Oversleeping or sleeping fewer than the recommended hours would lead to complications and irritation. Prolonged spans would lead to mental and physical complications and ailments.

- **Never stay up late** - Whatever needs to be done, ensure it is taken care of during your active hours. When the clock hits a specific time, pause everything, and go to sleep. You will need to religiously follow a sleeping pattern until it becomes a habit.

One of the greatest issues we face in today's world is not knowing when to put away our cell phones and tablets. While these may be a good source of entertainment and communication, they are not at all friendly to anyone who is trying to sleep. They emit a certain kind of ray that keeps our brains activated and constantly accepting information. While that happens, sleep eludes us, causing us to stay up late in the night. It is only when we put these electronic devices aside that we start to feel sleepy. If you suffer from such issues, turn your electronic devices off and retire to bed.

For anyone who may be suffering from insomnia or any other ailment, ensure that you check with a doctor for any medication or exercise that can help you to go to sleep.

Exercise, as discussed earlier, does greatly help everyone despite any ailment they may have. Through exercise, our body grows tired and naturally demands a good sleep. It is of no surprise then that those who sleep in the night after a hard day's work and a session at the gym feel far more relaxed than those who do not consider exercise as an option. Combining your love for exercise and your love for sleep will always allow you to reap some tremendous results. Fortunately, we need just that to lead a holistic life.

Nutrition

We cannot live without food. However, food is quite a broad term. Anything edible can be considered as food, but not all things edible are as essential or nourishing as others.

As human beings, we are easily distracted or tempted by various delicacies and food items. It is perfectly okay to have these, but relying solely on takeaway food, junk food, and oily food can lead to catastrophic consequences on our health. One significant consequence would see you gaining a chunk of weight in a very short span of time.

For the readers who may be quite slim and are looking to gain some extra pounds, I assure you this is not the kind of mass you wish to put on. These are mostly made up of bad fats, cholesterols, and other harmful ingredients. Instead, we should focus on following a diet plan that covers all the nutrients our body needs regularly.

The World Health Organization (WHO) describes that there are about six essential nutrients that should be made a part of your daily intake (Butler, 2018). Each one of these nutrients serves a significant purpose in ensuring a healthy body and maintaining healthy functions. If you have never looked at your diet seriously before, this is perhaps a good time to take in the information and analyze your daily diet.

1. **Protein** - It's not just about gaining mass; it serves as the building block for the body. Around 16% of our body is made up of protein (Butler, 2018), and that reinforces how important protein is. Some significant sources for protein are meat, fish, eggs, nuts, grains, and soy.

2. **Carbohydrates** - While the world is going insane behind the entire low-carb craze these days, one thing remains standing as a fact that cannot be overlooked: our bodies need carbohydrates. Depriving our bodies of carbs will never allow us to truly have a healthy body. With that said, however, you can undoubtedly take a controlled amount of carbohydrates, just about enough to maintain your physical health and not run into any complications. Some good sources of carbs are beans, whole-grain breads, fruits, and fiber-rich veggies.

3. **Fats** - Okay, I admit this might raise some eyebrows, but that is not anyone's fault. There are generally two types of fats, the good ones,

and the bad ones. Keep the latter away and consume the former. Fats, like omega-3, are super healthy for our bodies and allow for better mineral and vitamin absorption, muscle movement, and more. Fats do come packed with calories, and these calories serve as a vital source of fuel for the body to carry out its functions. Some great sources of healthy fats include nuts, fish, seeds, and certain vegetable oils. Avoid butter, red meat, and cheese.

4. **Vitamins** - Numerous vitamins are found in various food sources, but our body essentially needs 13 of these. The most important ones are vitamins A, B6, C, and D. Vitamins ensure that our body remains healthy and free from diseases and ailments. Vitamins are also crucial if you wish to maintain good skin, healthy vision, and some great hair and bones. Some great sources include meat, carrots, sweet potatoes, fish, seeds, nuts, and kale.

5. **Minerals** - These are almost the same in purpose as vitamins. They help our bodies remain healthy and continue to fight off ailments. They help our bodies carry out various functions as well. If you are to follow the sources I have listed above, you honestly do not need to look for any other types of food. Most of these will already provide you with the minerals you need.

6. **Water** - Ironic? Not at all. While water is available almost everywhere, we still have this baffling capacity of overlooking its importance. Without water, life as we know it would cease to exist. You can quite literally live for weeks without food, but you cannot make it to the end of a week without water. Simply put, water is our source of life. Consume the recommended eight glasses of water each day to ensure the smooth function of the body, brain, kidneys, and many more organs.

Balanced pH

Not many may know, but the natural state of a human body is alkaline in nature. While that is true, we continue to bombard our body with acidic content and food that upsets the scale and tilts the balance far too much to one side. This imbalance of the pH scale then paves the way for massive problems.

The perfect alkaline to acid ratio that we should try and aim for is 70:30. This is easier said than done as we usually never worry about what we are having to eat and whether it is acidic in nature or otherwise. So, why does this pH balance matter so much that we should start considering what we eat?

Quite a lot of bacteria, germs, diseases, and ailments thrive within acidic settings. If our acid levels are high, they have more room to mess around and damage our bodies from within. The higher the acidity, the more it is borrowed from our vital organs to try to neutralize the situation by removing the excess acid. Facing constant over-acidity damages our body and weakens it. The weaker our body, the more issues we face, such as chronic fatigue, candida issues, hormonal imbalance, and premature aging, which is quite a terrifying prospect for anyone. If I am to list down possible issues we humans can face owing to a pH imbalance, the list would be extensive and slightly worrying.

Fortunately, though, things are always looking brighter for those who wish to change their ways and take a healthier approach to life. It is never too late to begin, and perhaps now is your time to make this all-important change and feel the difference yourself.

The first order of the day would be to revisit your diet plan, if you have one. If not, simply start observing what you eat regularly. Certain food items fall under the acidic side of the pH scale while others naturally come under the alkaline side.

If you are looking for a bit of an easy way out, start avoiding processed flour and sugars, soda, most dairy products, tobacco, coffee (yes, you read that right), and some others. Try to find replacements that are healthier for you and provide you with energy without jeopardizing the remainder of your body.

There are tons of websites, blogs, and other useful resources that you can refer to and find the information suiting your specific needs, in case you are someone who suffers from issues like asthma and fatigue. For anyone already suffering from an imbalance, consult with your doctor at the earliest to minimize the damage. Some random tests may be done to further diagnose the issues you may be facing, followed by prescribed medication, which should effectively level out your pH balance.

Calm State of Mind

Perhaps the hardest thing by a country mile, there is no shortcut to achieving a truly calm and relaxed mind. Every second, our brain is processing massive amounts of data, and trying to calm it down automatically seems like an impossible task.

What people fail to understand is that our brain needs a bit of a time out. Sleep is one way to achieve this, but unless you know the code to unlock a blissful sleep, it will not do you much good. However, where there is a will, you will always find a way.

You can start with simple breathing exercises. These are great for calming your nerves and your mind when you face high levels of stress. There are various breathing exercises available on the internet, each with their own unique methods and results. Depending on what suits you, you can choose one and stick with it. Make it a daily thing and take the time to carry out the exercise for around 15 to 20 minutes every day. The results are fascinating, to say the least, and they genuinely make you feel more relaxed.

For a more long-term solution, start looking into meditation. Again, there are hundreds of techniques out there. Choosing one may be a bit tricky, but once you have found one that you are comfortable with, make the most of it by having a colleague, a friend, or your partner join in. Not only does it become a little social event, but all of the participants get to share their experiences and learn from one another. Meditation itself will help you to alleviate all your worries, stress, and anxiety. It greatly helps in managing your blood pressure if you suffer from high blood pressure.

Meditation also helps you learn how to focus your energy on one point. This is great, especially for people who find themselves distracted easily by noise of any kind. Through meditation, you can feel at peace, though it does take some time getting used to the postures and positions. It is a great way to reconnect with your soul, clear out your mind, and let your body heal naturally.

Other benefits include:

- Reduced stress
- Increased emotional regulation
- Increased resilience
- Improved physical well-being

- Increased empathy
- Increased respect
- Increased emotional intelligence

Slice it any way you would like, but that is quite a resume. It then makes it a no-brainer; meditation is indeed an answer that has always been there for us. The calmer your mind is, the more productive your day will be.

Spiritual Practices

At first, I was a little skeptical on this front. There is a common misunderstanding that spiritual practices center around being religious, praying, worshipping, and being engaged in such activities. The fact of the matter is that these are indeed ways to connect to your spirituality, but they are not the only ways to do so.

This perhaps would be an ideal time to give you one piece of good news. If you have followed the book so far, you have already discovered one of the most significant ways to connect to your spirit and feel alive again. Meditation is the primary choice for hundreds and thousands of people who wish to further strengthen their spirituality, discover their mantras, and harness the power of chi from within. Add that to any religious activities, such as prayers and rituals, and you are already set to have this aspect of yourself covered.

As an additional measure, incorporate the habit of giving to others. If you have unnecessary things lying around, consider donating those to people who may need them more than you. Not only does it help to declutter, but it makes you feel happy from within. Your soul feels redeemed, knowing that you were able to give something back to the community. It is a feeling that has worked for many cases. It is one of the most beautiful ways to not only set an example within society, but also to feel spiritually elevated to new heights.

Being Emotionally Expressive

One of the biggest hurdles we face in the kind of world we live in is to express our honest opinions and emotions. There are far too many factors that push us into an uncomfortable zone where we cannot show our emotions properly, fearing that doing so will have us labeled as *an emotional freak*. We quickly get used to this, learn how to hide our emotions, and believe that is that; you might want to think again.

Hiding emotions is okay at times, but not always. Imagine that your mind and body are like a balloon. It can certainly hold some air in, but too much of it, and we, just like the balloon, will burst. All that emotion we once managed to hide will now flow out waywardly and end up hurting quite a few people while raising a lot of eyebrows. And that is not the end of it either, because as soon as you experience one of these outbursts, you are immediately asked to visit a psychiatrist or a professional healer. That is more money steaming out of your account.

Learning how to handle our emotions and responding to situations appropriately definitely helps us in life. Not only does it allow us to express our emotions properly, without causing too much trouble, but it certainly adds to our wellbeing.

Ever felt like you needed to cry your heart out or just scream out loud? That happens to most of us, and the culprit here is not being emotionally expressive. Had we expressed our emotions properly and at the right time, we would have never felt these instances of buildup in the first place.

There is a reason why some of the most successful people remain calm and composed every single day. They have learned and mastered the art of being emotionally intelligent. Just like the intelligence quotient (IQ), everyone also has what is called emotional intelligence (EQ). This is the ability of a person to recognize their own emotions and the emotions of those around them. The higher the EQ, the better they understand and react to given situations. The lower the EQ, the more irritated, angry, and rude they tend to get.

A good EQ helps us to communicate better with others and understand just how they might respond. It also helps us learn how to react to given situations. For example, a noise in the dark might scare some away. Some may find it attractive and hence explore the source. Regardless of which one you may be, you need to know what situations cause you to have fits of rage or make you feel like you are emotionally breaking down. Once identified, you can work on these situations to master them and learn how to respond correctly. Eventually, when you know what needs to be done at any given situation, you can throw your emotions into the mix and efficiently use those to describe how you feel and what should be done without losing your temper, your nerves, or giving into fear.

Remember, the more you express, the better you start to feel about yourself. And yes, if that means you need to be honest with someone about a dress they bought that clearly does not suit them, let them know. There is a fine line between being honest and being rude. Had you screamed or yelled or even insulted the other person's choice with words like, "Are you blind? Can you not see how that makes you look ugly?", would have been downright rude. Avoid rude remarks and stick to honesty. It will eventually save you from a lot of hassle. Lastly, being expressive is always good for health and reduces the chances of suffering issues like fits, strokes, heart attacks, high blood pressure, and so on.

Why Should I Pursue Such a Lifestyle?

This is a reasonably good question. You might be overwhelmed already just by going through the previous section, but I assure you one thing: the fruits of all these changes are far greater than you might imagine.

This holistic lifestyle, when combined with the above habits and tips, brings forth the finest person within you, out of the darkness and into the light. This confident, peaceful, and charming person would automatically start gaining some attention. When you work on yourself, your mind, body, and soul, there is absolutely nothing that will stand in the way of you and your success.

With a renewed spirit, a more focused mind, and a body that is ready to take on the challenges of the day, you would be gearing up for a very different and exciting life compared to the one you have been living so far. Everything would now seem achievable because you know you have what it takes to make that possible. This kind of lifestyle comes loaded with some other perks, which are long-lasting and continue to add a charm to your life in one way or another.

Longevity

Exercising regularly and having a holistic approach means that you are paying attention to all your needs, whether physical, emotional, or spiritual. A happier person would always end up living longer than an unhappy one.

Increased Mental and Physical Performance

Whether you aim to lead an organization, display your athleticism, take part in endurance contests, or impress your partner in bed, performance is the key element. Through the holistic ways, you are always confident, knowing that you have all the abilities to get the job done to perfection. The difference would be significant, so much so that you and those around you will notice and admire it.

Increased Happiness

Unlocking the key to eternal happiness is perhaps a lifelong dream; however, through the holistic lifestyle, you can undoubtedly acquire just that. By knowing how to care for your body, mind, and soul, there is almost nothing that would feel left out or ignored. You would always wake up happy and sleep even more satisfied, knowing that you had a great day.

Freedom

Being emotionally expressive and confident, you would soon start to feel as free as a bird. You can do whatever you like because you are doing it for your own sake. Where you once were not able to express your emotions or share your opinion, you would now be making an impression and expressing your true feelings like never before.

Freedom isn't just about having enough money, it is far more than that. It is a mental state where you get to choose what you wish to do, whom you want to speak with, and how you would like to spend the rest of your day. That can only be made possible if you have a mind, a body, and a soul that is capable of handling daily issues and converting them into opportunities. By blocking the negativity, you would always be seeking the brighter side of things, and that would ultimately lead to the success you never knew existed. That is true freedom, and now you know just how to get it.

How to Get Started Then?

Well, there are a few ways you can do so. I had already listed some earlier, but to get you up to speed, hit the gym as soon as you can. Thinking about it will never do you much good. The real fruit lies within an action that you need to take.

Take the first step and know you are a step closer to your goal already. Focus on your food consumption and keep check on how balanced your diet is. Ensure that you speak to a trainer, as that dramatically helps at the gym if you are someone who has no idea what kind of exercises you need to do. If that doesn't tickle your fancy, how about jumping straight to the good old

ACV? After all, this book primarily focuses on apple cider vinegar.

If the above has confused you, I assure you that the next chapter will clear out any doubts you may be having. Holistic lifestyle is indeed something to pursue, but there are far too many things which do tend to get in the way, such as keeping an eye on your diet. You cannot do that every single time, and that is where the ACV comes in. Consider it as a shortcut, and with that in mind, let us dive into the next chapter and start discovering just how ACV can help us achieve what we are looking for.

Chapter 2:

The Science Behind Apple Cider Vinegar

In the last chapter, we looked at holistic living, a lifestyle that promotes one to discover and understand their physical, mental, and spiritual side. It is one of the most effective methods of leading a healthy lifestyle, and the rewards are certainly worth the effort. With that said, let us further explore why I termed apple cider vinegar as a shortcut.

I intend to stay true to my words and further explain just what ACV is, how incredibly beneficial it is, and why you should opt to add ACV to your regular diet routine. This chapter, then, will explore all these fronts and bring forth all the details one should know before proceeding into this astonishing world of benefits.

We will look into the science that lies behind apple cider vinegar. We will have a detailed look into what makes ACV such a great hit with the masses and analyze whether ACV lives up to its reputation. We shall also be looking into a quick recipe and learn how to make our very own ACV at home, and how much of it you should consume. All that is to come, and there is no better way to start than to answer the burning question many may have, especially the ones who are entirely new to apple cider vinegar.

What Is Apple Cider Vinegar?

In the most basic terms, ACV is nothing more than fermented apples and water. It is a simple home-made remedy that has gone on to claim the status of 'superfood' owing to the various benefits it brings to the table.

It is straightforward to make, and it does not need refrigeration at all. As long as you keep it at room temperature, it should be perfectly fine to consume. If that wasn't enough, ACV has an extremely long shelf life. That means you can make one batch and use it for a very, very long time. This is because almost every type of vinegar, in its natural form, has an indefinite shelf life. ACV, being a product of apples and vinegar, carries the torch forward.

ACV has existed for quite some time, but it has only made a global impact in the last few years. With millions of people using ACV to cut down on weight and treat various diseases, it is of no surprise that it has garnered the attention of the world. Nowadays, almost every other person wants in on the action and is looking to use ACV for various purposes, most commonly weight loss.

Regardless of the purpose you intend to use ACV for, it is quite beneficial and can certainly add flavor to your food without jeopardizing the calorie count.

The Science Behind It

Vinegar, derived from the French words *vin* and *aigre*, simply means *sour vine*. Owing to the presence of acetic acid, the vinegar tastes sour. Apple cider vinegar is made by allowing apples to be broken down by yeast. The yeast completely digests all the sugar contents within the apple and breaks them down into alcohol. Once that is done, the naturally occurring bacteria, called acetobacter, then convert this alcohol into acetic acid. This process is called fermentation. We will dive into details later on where we will learn just how we can make our very own batch of ACV.

ACV is rich in polyphenols and B-vitamins, just like the apple juice itself. This then makes ACV a nutrient-rich and tasty drink. There have been numerous studies that have been conducted, and some of these have shown significant benefits to health. Some of these health benefits are:

- **Blood Sugar Level Control** - If you are someone who needs to monitor their blood sugar level on and off, I am happy to report that ACV dramatically helps you in maintaining the right blood sugar level. A study published by the American Diabetes Association in 2004 detailed encouraging findings (Butler, 2019). A select few participants were provided with ACV, the others being given a placebo, after consumption of butter, orange juice, and a bagel. The participants who consumed 20 grams of ACV showed significantly lower blood sugar levels after the meal.

- **ACV Fights Bacteria on Your Salads** - A few drops of ACV on your favorite salad will stop the bacterial growth and leave your salad fresh, with a bit of added flavor.

- **ACV Helps in Weight Loss** - This is possibly the most significant reason behind the hype of ACV. Yes, it does help in weight loss, but it is to be made clear that ACV alone cannot do anything. Couple that with an active routine and exercise, and the results will astonish you.

- **Diluted ACV Helps Fight Acne Problems** - Owing to the nature of vinegar, and the acetic acid present within it, a diluted form of ACV can be an excellent asset for those looking for acne-related treatments.

- **Restores Scalp pH** - While we covered the importance of a balanced pH level within our body, the scalp can quickly lose its pH balance through the application of various shampoos. Most shampoos have a higher alkaline property, which can lead to a dry and irritated scalp. This means you are more likely to suffer from hair loss and frizzy hair. ACV counterbalances the shampoo with its acidic nature, leaving you with a healthy scalp and strengthened hair. It is also a great way to stop hair loss.

To summarize things, vinegar, or the sour vine, greatly helps in fighting off unwanted bacteria and allows us to feel better, fresher, and healthier. While the internet covers an array of benefits, I intend to cover the ones which are proven either through research or personal experience.

With that said, it is now time to get our feet wet and learn how to make our very own batch of apple cider vinegar. After all, there is no point in reading about ACV unless you aim to try it out yourself.

Making Your Very Own ACV

The recipe to make a batch of apple cider vinegar is quite simple. It does not require you to buy anything unusually expensive nor to look for special ingredients. To make the most of your purchase, or products, ensure you use every bit of it. That means, even the scraps can be used to create an effective batch of apple cider vinegar. The scraps include the apple core and the skin.

During the process, you will come across a rather unusual layer of a cloudy substance that floats around.

This is generally seen when making ACV at home, as it is raw, unpasteurized, and unfiltered. Do not be alarmed by that or rush to remove it. It's quite useful. It is called "mother," and it is formed naturally and eventually settles at the bottom of the bottle.

Things You Need to Get Started

Grab a pen, or use your phone to note these down. You must get the recipe right as tiny details can often change the end results.

1. **A Clean Jar** - When I say clean, I mean crystal clear. You can pick up any jar you would like or go for a trusty old wide-mouth quart jar.

2. **Natural Apple Scraps** - The core, the peels, even the slices if you choose, though I prefer to consume the slices and only use the scraps. The quantity should be just enough to fill 3/4 of the jar.

3. **Cane Sugar** - Organic, two tablespoons

4. **Water** - Unchlorinated and filtered, two cups

5. **Filter** - A cheesecloth or a coffee filter should do the trick

6. **Rubber Band** - To tie the cloth around the mouth of the jar

7. **Fermentation Weight** - A separate small jar or any other kind of fermentation weight that can help keep the apples below the water level

For those interested in taking a peek at the calorie count and the time it takes, here is a little additional information:

Prep Time - 5 minutes

Servings - Around 18 servings (15-30 grams per serving)

Calories/serving - 6

Okay, I do admit the total time is a little tricky to gauge. Some claim it can take two weeks, and then others claim it takes a total of 40 days. However, I will cover the basics here and all that you need to know to identify when your ACV batch is ready. Let us now begin with the process.

Instructions

1. Clean your empty jar and let it air dry completely.

2. Fill the jar with apple scraps until it is filled 3/4 of the way. For those who might be using whole apples, chop them up before putting them into the jar.

3. Mix and dissolve the cane sugar into the cup of water.

4. Pour the sugar water into the jar with the apples. The point here is to ensure that the apples are completely submerged. You can add additional water as well, if needed to fully immerse them.

5. Use the fermentation weight to ensure all apples are below the water level. This is mandatory as any apple exposed to air might grow mold, and that can ruin the batch.

6. Cover the mouth of the jar with your cheesecloth or coffee filter. Use the rubber band to secure the cloth in position.

7. Store the jar in a dark place at room temperature. You will need to store it for at least three weeks.

8. It is best to check on the jar daily. Check for any mold. If all is well, give it a quick stir, cover the lid once again, and put it back into its place. Continue this every day or at least three times a week.

9. Keep an eye out for bubble formation. That is a sign indicating the process is going smoothly.

10. After about three weeks, the solution should smell sweet. At this point, strain the apple

pieces out of the solution and compost them. Return the liquid into the jar and keep it stored.

11. Now, it is all about acquiring the right taste. Keep checking by tasting it every day to see when it feels right to you. Once there, simply transfer the contents to another jar, and your ACV is ready to be used.

But wait, where's the mother I spoke of? When you are straining the apples, keep an eye out for the cloudy floating substance. That is essentially the mother I was referring to. At times, it floats at the top, like a gelatinous layer, while in other instances, it may settle at the bottom of the jar.

Hello Mother!

The mother is a stringy, gelatinous substance made up of all that is good for us. It contains dozens of useful bacteria. These are often referred to as probiotics, and these help us in maintaining a perfectly functioning digestive system. The healthier our digestive system, the better we harness all the goodness from the food we consume.

Probiotics are generally beneficial as they help in strengthening our immune system. Surprisingly, most of these are located within our digestive tract, which makes the mother even more useful. I will discuss the details in the next chapter to further shed light on how these actually help in doing what they do.

Since we are talking about digestive systems, I should also point out that the mother comes packed with enzymes that play a significant role in breaking down food and allowing our body to consume the nutrients from them.

Now comes the part on how to use ACV with the mother, and this is important to know. Get this wrong, and you might end up facing some nasty side-effects.

How Much to Consume?

Your consumption of the raw ACV, with or without the mother, should be diluted with some water. This is something you honestly would want to do as the acidity levels in the raw ACV can harm your tooth enamel. Also, the diluted solution should be limited to one to a maximum of two tablespoons per day.

If your jar contains the mother floating within, shake the jar well before use. This ensures that the solution contains some essential bits which further help in strengthening your digestive system and in controlling your blood sugar levels.

Ideally, you would want to start with small amounts. Half a teaspoon should be enough to get you acquainted with the taste and develop a taste for it as you go along. Once you see some results, you can increase the intake to a full teaspoon. Eventually, it is your call whether you would like to up the dose to two teaspoons or stay at one. Care must be taken not to exceed the maximum dose per day. This can certainly bring harmful results, and we are trying everything possible to avoid those.

Now that you know how to make your very own batch of ACV, and you know about the intake and the mother as well, it is time to shift gears and step into a more practical aspect: detoxing the body. Whether you aim to lose weight or discover any other benefit covered by ACV, prepare yourself to take some notes and pointers. We have quite a lot to learn and even more to experience in the next chapter.

Chapter 3:

It's Time to Detox

If you have just made it here, you may remember that I mentioned I would be discussing in detail about how probiotics work. As promised, this chapter will primarily focus on how exactly these probiotics work, how they help with detoxification, and so much more.

When we talk about detoxification, there are quite a lot of elements that come into play. Some are trying to detox their bodies from harmful chemicals and substances stuck within their digestive tracts, while others are merely trying something to further help them shed some weight. Either way, detoxification is a process that takes some time before any visible changes can be seen and felt.

Similarly, using ACV as your detox method should not be expected to show significant results overnight. It takes time, commitment, and consistency to ensure that the true nature of ACV and the benefits it brings can manifest.

I have already given you a small peek into some of the most commonly reported benefits. Truth be told, they alone are quite remarkable. While the world of science continues to study the ACV hype further, no one can deny that it genuinely helps us and our body to feel better.

If you have already started working towards a holistic lifestyle, as we discussed in the first chapter, it should make more sense now as to why ACV is so essential. We can take care of our bodies, but that's mostly limited to external factors such as our appearance, hygiene, and clothing. What goes on inside our bodies, we can do little to control that. By using ACV, we are now allowing our bodies to get the care they deserve. By flushing out all that is harmful and, in a way, cleansing our bodies, we ensure everything inside remains healthy day in and day out.

How ACV Helps with Detox

Apple cider vinegar boasts quite a few benefits for the blood and skin. It serves as a healing agent and contains detoxification properties that help our digestive system, particularly our liver. Our liver, if bogged down with bacteria or other harmful substances, can cause quite a lot of issues for the body. Using ACV ensures that our liver is flushed and, as a result, allows an improved blood filtration process. Pure blood means more energy for the body.

When using diluted ACV, you can throw in a pinch of sugar or honey to further amp up the taste. As an added measure, drink plenty of water to aid the detoxification process.

In the previous chapter, we discussed how the mother comes packed with enzymes. These enzymes are vital in ensuring a smooth detoxification process. These enzymes come into action by attacking the toxins within our body. By doing so, these toxins are eventually forced out of our systems, leaving behind a healthier liver and digestive tract.

ACV contains some good bacteria, which I am sure you already know by now. However, the purpose of having these good bacteria is to strike a healthy balance within our system. How? Let's look at a microscopic level and see what is what.

Equalizes Bacterial Balance

Our colon and digestive tract contain most of the bacteria found within our bodies. These are naturally occurring, which often misleads people into thinking all of them are good. The natural balance would be 80% good bacteria and 20% bad bacteria. This figure is quite important. A rise in the bad bacteria would see us getting sick almost instantly.

Good bacteria work by competing for all the available resources with the bad bacteria. The higher the number of good bacteria, the more resources they can gather for good use. The bad bacteria, on the other hand, are always out to create a mess that can cause ailment and diseases.

ACV, packed with the good bacteria, provides a fresh supply to our body and helps in correcting and maintaining that balance we may have lost over time.

Immune System Booster

Naturally, when ACV is doing its job and is doing it rather well, it does boost your overall immune system. By flushing out all the toxins, promoting a healthy digestive system, and providing a balance of the good bacteria against the bad, there is little to question the claim that ACV helps in strengthening your immune system.

With that said, however, relying only on ACV might not do the trick for you. You need to ensure that you continue to opt for a healthy diet, one that consists of green vegetables. They are one of the finest sources to provide your body the boost it needs to ramp up your immune system. Add that to the fact that the probiotics in ACV hold an immune-boosting effect, which works like a charm and allows your body to fight off most viruses and ailments. For anyone suffering from a cold or the flu, ACV usage can greatly shorten the duration of the ailment.

Detox for Skin

This has indeed captured the eyes and minds of many ACV fans around the world. While ACV is primarily used as food intake, it can also be applied topically to help what is effectively termed as the third kidney of the human body — our skin.

For those who may not be familiar with the medical aspect, let me give you a brief explanation about what exactly the skin does. This would then clarify just how important of a role ACV has for our skin.

Our skin is the largest organ in existence. It is constantly working, day and night, to excrete about one-third of the waste material from the skin directly. Our sweat causes quite a lot of detoxification, which is eventually thrown out of our bodies. Sometimes, it leads to acne problems, while others may end up with dried skin. This usually happens for several reasons, chief among them being an unbalanced pH level.

ACV can be applied topically to skin pores by gently massaging it. It gets absorbed rather easily and hence removes all the clogs, ultimately reducing the acne. With repeated use, you will start to notice a fresher, more radiant-looking skin. It will be softer and smoother, as well.

You can quite literally say goodbye to the expensive makeup materials and treatments because you now have everything you need to get that glowing skin, right in your kitchen.

Another amazing feature of ACV is that it provides our skin with almost 40 minerals, vitamins, and those good enzymes. They greatly help in detoxifying, healing, nourishing, replenishing, and protecting the skin from harm. No wonder there are communities online that continue to post terrific results and application methods every single day.

There are far too many benefits for the skin when it comes to ACV. Whenever I get to talk about ACV and the numerous benefits it has for the skin, quite a lot of people pay extra attention, and rightly so. Therefore, I promise you, we will look into the skin aspect with a lot more detail later in the book. Covering this aspect in just a few paragraphs would be unjust.

ACV as Diuretics

It is what it sounds like. Diuretics can be any substance that promotes and boosts the production of urine from the body. The more we urinate, the more we flush out all the toxins and unwanted substances from our bodies. Consider this as a natural filter that discards everything that can potentially harm us from within.

With that said, however, some find it hard to pass urine frequently or may not notice that their urine production is less than that of an average person. This can be rather alarming and can have dire consequences for our health.

Fortunately, ACV is here to help as it dramatically helps in promoting the production of urine. Why? It's simply because vinegar is a natural diuretic option and has been known to boost the production of urine to flush the system out. While it does that, it comes with an added benefit. It can prevent potassium-depleting effects, which are generally associated with diuretics, natural or otherwise.

This, coupled with a strengthened digestive system, further helps in digesting all the food from the last day, which otherwise would leave you feeling sluggish and down. All you need is to ensure a bit of consistency, and the rest is just magic.

Blocks Growth of Certain Types of Cancer Cells

This is certainly a big one. There have been studies where ACV's potential cancer healing properties were put to the test. Astonishingly, it showed that it was able to kill off the gastric cancer cells. That is quite a surprising feat for something that has been both criticized and ridiculed without proper research. After this finding, further research is underway to find out just how effective and applicable this can be (Cafasso, 2018).

How you take this up is absolutely your call, but one thing is sure; if there is even the slightest truth in it, I am sure this is going to change the world as we know it.

ACV Looks Promising!

Needless to say, with so many benefits, ACV is looking like a true competitor, one that just might be able to save the day for hundreds of thousands of people around the globe. It is cheap, it is viable, it is feasible, and above all, it tastes nice. There is almost no reason why one should not include ACV in their regular intake unless they genuinely hate the taste of it.

It is one of the most effective detoxification methods. Other ways would see you drink bitter juices and use costly medications. This, on the other hand, is none of those. I assure you that once you see the benefits yourself, it is quite hard to look the other way.

Sure, there are studies and websites which still continue to oppose the entire concept of ACV. Sure enough, you would find many more who would be more than happy to provide their criticism, despite never having tried ACV themselves. This is but natural; opinions will always exist. It is entirely your call on how you perceive ACV and what exactly your goals are which you wish to achieve through the use of ACV.

I do recommend that you know your goals clearly and that they are realistic in nature. You cannot start using ACV and expect to lose 20 pounds within a week. The only way that might be possible would be to starve yourself to near death, and that is the polar opposite of what we are trying to do here.

Lastly, before we jump to our next chapter, I do wish to clarify that you do not need to have a few extra pounds on you to try ACV for yourself. As long as you have the will to lead a life where you are fit physically, mentally, and spiritually, you can enjoy the rich benefits of apple cider vinegar just as much as anyone else.

In the next chapter, we will be switching our attention away from detox and see just how the apple cider vinegar helps us in keeping our heart healthy. Not too long ago, I briefly mentioned that ACV helps in maintaining our blood sugar levels. We will now cover that in great detail to truly understand just how it manages to do so.

Chapter 4:

Enhanced Heart Health and Lowered Blood Sugar

One of the most alarming health hazards the people of the world face these days relates to our heart. Our heart is the most important organ within our body. Its function isn't just to beat and keep the blood flowing at a steady pace, but it is far more than that. If anything was to hamper the heartbeat, or if the heart was to skip just a single beat, it could lead us into a world of serious trouble and agony.

Despite its importance, we humans have developed this incredible ability to overlook its care. If we were to come with instructions, our heart would certainly have a "handle with care" sticker on it. The rest of the body would do just fine, but the heart needs extra special care.

Statistics show just how grim the situation has become in recent years. Just within the United States, heart disease is named the leading cause of death. Every 37 seconds, a person dies in the US due to cardiovascular disease. That is a staggering 647,000 deaths a year, all because of heart disease (CDC, 2019). If we do the math correctly, that comes up to one of every four deaths, and that is beyond an alarming situation. Financially speaking, heart disease costs the US around $219 billion a year, and that was just from 2014 to 2015. We are now in the year 2020, and if anything, that number would have certainly increased.

With such a high number of fatalities, it makes more sense to seek out alternatives that can help us keep our hearts healthy and away from all the potential risks involved. Exercising is one way, but that alone is not enough. It has less to do with the exercise itself and more to do with the fact that we cannot devote much time to exercise as we always have other commitments to worry about.

If that wasn't grim enough for you, here is another statistic about yet another issue that has plagued the people of the world: diabetes.

The Center for Disease Control and Prevention has come to a conclusion that highlights some of the leading causes of heart disease, and diabetes stands right at the top. In 2018, a study was conducted by the American Diabetes Association, and it showed a shockingly high number of diabetes patients within the US alone. Around 34.2 million people within the US suffered from diabetes. That is 10.5% of the total population of the country, and whichever way you look at it, it is a massive number.

Clearly, there is something at play here that is causing these diseases to spread in such a dramatic way. I am not going to fall for the so-called theories we keep hearing about from the propaganda specialists as I genuinely believe in statistics and facts. However, the facts indicate that we pay little attention to the type of foods we eat and rarely take exercise as seriously as it should be considered.

If you are someone who consumes quite a lot of oily, fatty, and possibly fried food items, such as chips, fries, or chicken nuggets, stop immediately. Unless you are 100% sure that the food is being prepared in an omega-3 rich oil, it is time to put a pause on your habits and take some time to allow your body to recover its lost energy and health.

Typically, at this point, people would rush to their nearest herbal medicine stores and hope to find some kind of herbal mixture that could help them recover from any damage that might have been done. Fortunately, you do not need to do that at all. At least now, you are already familiar with an effective method that can help you in your path to recovery.

Using ACV regularly would allow you to not only look better, but it will promote your heart's health and lower blood sugar levels, as well. You will genuinely feel the renewed energy within you, allowing you to do more than you could have done before.

In this chapter, we will look in detail at how ACV will help us fight off heart disease and revive its health, and we will also shed some light on how exactly it helps in keeping our blood sugar levels low.

ACV for the Heart

Apple cider vinegar is known for numerous benefits, but one of the leading benefits it has to offer is related to the heart. Multiple factors contribute to an increase or a decrease in the heart's health. ACV steps in to provide a much-needed balance and support in cleaning out our systems effectively.

For those who may not be familiar with heart complications, the most common issue we have is high cholesterol. Imagine a pipe that transports water from one end to the other. As long as the pipe is clear and has no obstructions, the water should flow smoothly and without any issues. Once the pipe starts to clog, the flow rate of water will change. The more the pipe clogs up with debris and dirt, the narrower the passage will be for water to go through. This means that as water goes through this passage, it will increase the pressure significantly. The pipe might be able to handle significant pressure, but the same concept does not apply to the human heart.

Similar to the clogging of the pipe, our vessels and arteries, which are connected to the heart, get clogged by cholesterol deposits. Naturally, almost all of us have some cholesterol in our body, but it is what we eat that either adds to the cholesterol or cleans it.

A choked blood vessel or artery will start to create pressure on the heart. As a result, the heart will need to exert more pressure in order to deal with the change and will have to beat faster to continue a smooth supply of oxygenated blood. A raised heart rate is okay for brief periods, but if left unchecked, or if the heart continues to beat faster than usual, then it is time to put everything aside and rush to the hospital.

Apple cider vinegar can significantly help by lowering cholesterol levels. Initial tests show promising signs. Those who have used apple cider vinegar continue to sing songs of praise as well.

In an ideal world, you would be avoiding several food items to ensure that your cholesterol levels never shoot up or go wild. However, it is never too late to make that change. Here are some of the culprits which can certainly take a toll on your heart's health by throwing quite a lot of cholesterol your way:

- Processed red meat
- Soda
- Trans fats
- Fried food
- White bread
- Rice

- Pasta
- Breakfast cereal
- Fast food
- Butter

If you can manage to avoid these altogether, bravo! If not, you can start by lowering their consumption while starting with ACV at the same time.

Apart from the cholesterol levels, ACV also helps in lowering triglyceride levels and does the same for many other risk factors as well (Marengo, 2018).

Another culprit behind heart attacks and diseases is elevated blood pressure. This is a common ailment suffered by many. Using ACV in your regular diet can help prevent such issues. By lowering the blood pressure, you are effectively taking away two of the most significant contributors known to cause heart issues.

There have been other sources and reviews which have gone on to claim that apple cider vinegar can actually treat a range of heart diseases (*Therapeutic Effects of Vinegar: A Review*, 2019). For those who may not know, there is more than just a single heart disease out there, and that makes ACV quite something.

The Benefits of Having a Healthy Heart

A healthy heart can make a profound difference in anyone's life. It goes without saying that having a healthy heart allows you to do so much more, but, unfortunately, we take things for granted. We don't appreciate the fact that we may have a healthy lifestyle and a heart that is functioning perfectly. It is only when we run into these diseases and ailments that we realize just how wrong we were. It is then where we start looking at others, wondering how fortunate they are for not suffering these ailments.

Not so long ago, I had an opportunity to be a part of a discussion where the benefits of a healthy heart were brought up. Sometimes, we are often met with situations where we end up saying, "Duh! Everyone knows that!" I felt exactly the same way, right until I decided to check my own knowledge.

I tried to list down the benefits I thought I knew, and I ended with a list that contained only three entries. Why? Because we do have this nasty habit of taking everything for granted and thinking we know it all. We automatically start assuming that we know all the possible pros and cons. That may be vaguely correct, but when asked to define each one of them, we fail miserably and end up embarrassing ourselves.

Luckily, you do not have to go through that ordeal some of us may have faced by now. An even better news is that the benefits of questions are actually worth knowing. Provided that you pay close attention to your heart's health, you can reap tons of benefits in the years to come.

Caring for your heart and avoiding unnecessary cholesterol intake, smoking, or anything remotely dangerous can allow your heart to recover from any damage it may have faced. Of course, there are certain types of damages which might require medical procedures and surgeries, but for this book only, we will leave those dire situations out.

If you are someone who is in their 20s, good news! If you start working on your heart's health and maintain a healthy heart throughout your 20s, you will have a better functioning brain in middle age. The heart pumps blood throughout our body, and the mind is one of the most vital components that need blood. With an abrupt or hampered blood supply, we will most likely end up grumpy, with headaches, migraines, and many other disturbing issues.

A study conducted in 2017, which also appeared within the journal, *Neurology*, proves exactly the same thing. The results were conclusive and irrefutable in nature. Over the course of 30 years, 518 people were observed and closely studied. The study began when the subjects were in their 20s, and their heart readings and measurements were recorded. After every 2 to 5 years, they were subjected to various scans and tests, including tests on the brain as well. For 25 years, this went on, and data was gathered until the results were evidently clear.

A larger brain is attributed to a healthier heart. Those whose brain shrunk showed lower cognitive function scores, and they were more prone to strokes from the rest (*How a Healthy Heart Can Benefit Your Brain*, 2018).

After reading that, the readers who are 30 years old or more might be wondering if they missed their window. I am happy to report that you still have time to do something. Yes, you might not be able to enjoy exactly the same condition, but you can certainly be near. ACV is one of the most effective ways to maintain good health when it comes to the heart. Use ACV in recommended doses, and you should soon be flushing out all the unnecessary waste and toxins within your body while also lowering the cholesterol levels.

Another study, published in 2017 by JAMA research, showed that the very same people who were prone to suffering from a stroke or other heart conditions were also likely to develop unpleasant changes within their brains. I am not talking about shrinking or expanding the size of the brain. No, I am indeed referring to changes that can lead a person into the terrifying domain of Alzheimer's disease.

The study comprised a group of 346 people aged 50-59. They had no history of dementia. After nearly 25 years in the study, the results of various scans were in, and they were anything but encouraging. A massive 61% of the people who suffered from some cardiovascular issues from middle-age showed the development of amyloid protein fragments, which is what leads to

Alzheimer's disease (*How a Healthy Heart Can Benefit Your Brain,* 2018).

Right about now, you might be wondering what exactly we can do to avoid all this. I have already given you an idea on how ACV can help, but there are a few more things which I would recommend you do:

- **Stop Smoking** - You have heard this a million times already, but I assure you it is still as dangerous. Quit smoking as soon as you can. It is only the first few weeks which might cause a bit of discomfort, but once you get past that, you will never look back at another cigarette again.

- **Start Exercising** - Exercise is the answer to many issues, ailments, and diseases. Exercising helps us strengthen our muscles, and that includes the heart muscles as well. With a stronger heart muscle, our heart works more effectively.

- **Reduce Your Weight** - An increased weight means more work for our heart. Our heart can only pump blood to a certain level. The more we burden it, the higher the chance of heart issues. By reducing your weight, you are reducing that excess burden.

- **Change Your Diet** - Stop with oily food. Stop junk food and, most certainly, stop fast food.

Eat healthy, drink healthy, and the rest should work just like a charm. Holistic living or otherwise, a healthy diet is far more important than given credit.

- **Manage Your Blood Pressure** - Keep a few breathing exercises with yourself and use them to lower your stress levels and blood pressure.

These alone are enough measures for anyone to know of and follow. The results will surely come along the way. It is now time to move on to the second issue at hand: blood sugar level.

Controlling Your Blood Sugar Level

I already shared that grim-sounding research a few pages ago. It is a report that should leave anyone stunned, shocked, and rather worried. It is only natural you feel that way as there is a good chance a little miscalculation might put you in harm's way. If anything, we are trying to avoid just that.

My goal is to provide you with enough information that is both reliable and result-oriented. How you choose to apply it is your call, but I honestly cannot urge you enough to try it out and feel the difference.

Blood sugar levels within a healthy person vary in a controlled manner. When we wake up in the morning, they are somewhere between 70 to 100 mg/dL. Anything below that is alarming, and anything above that is equally as threatening. While there are fewer cases of those who may suffer from low blood sugar levels, the most reported cases of diabetic patients show an upward trend.

The healthy range is under 140mg/dL two hours after a meal. This is usually where things go wrong for most diabetic patients. Those who are diagnosed are already keeping an eye on their sugar levels, but the ones who are yet to know or be diagnosed with diabetes have no clue.

I know people who would end up with sugar levels through the roof--I am talking about levels exceeding 350mg/dL--and that is serious enough to get you hospitalized. Anything above the normal range can be a cause of worry. While there is injectable insulin, it can only do so much and is often limited. Get the dose wrong, and your sugar level can take a nosedive and go below 100mg/dL only an hour or so after a meal, and that too is dangerous.

A question then arises: why do we need to keep a balanced blood sugar level? The answer is rather easy. Our body is made up of cells, and sugar serves as a source of energy for these cells. Get it too high, and they get clogged up, shut down, and stop functioning. Get the levels too low, and they do not have enough energy to work correctly. Either of these situations would cause your naturally occurring insulin to take a hit.

This is often why you may see people suffering from headaches, body aches, joint pain, and even collapsing when their blood sugar levels spike up or down. This is a fairly common sight these days, unfortunately, and yet people remain unaware of it.

These uncontrollable sugar levels can cause a considerable amount of distress, pain, lethargy, and anxiety. If these are not controlled within time, things can get rather ugly and expensive, too. Diabetes is known to cause fatalities, and that also is a massive number. But why is this number rising day by day?

There was a time when we used to eat food that consisted of highly complex carbohydrates. Those took a reasonably long time to break down within our intestines, some of what we ate converted to vinegar before being absorbed. This would have triggered a signal, and our body would have released insulin on demand. Now, with so much processed food on the market, the carbohydrates are highly refined. This translates to food that is absorbed within our bodies well before being broken down properly, and that means our body never gets the signal to produce insulin. No insulin means the sugar levels in our blood will soar higher.

The insulin injections are certainly an option to counter that. However, if you're someone who has a bit of a phobia of needles, relax; ACV is here to save the day. That is one solid reason for you to start using ACV and avoid ever getting caught in a place where you are stuck with a needle to inject a dose of insulin into your body.

According to research conducted by Arizona State University (Spero, 2018), a few subjects were asked to drink 20 grams of ACV, 40 grams of water, and 1 teaspoon of saccharin with each meal. The results showed that the ones who used ACV had 34% lower blood sugar levels after the meal compared to the ones who were using other methods to control their blood sugar levels.

Such a fantastic result, and yet most diabetic patients either refuse to take it or have no idea about its potential power. It is termed as "the most cost-effective medicine" in history.

ACV, when consumed, triggers the necessary response and allows our body to produce insulin and other hormones to ensure they do not miss out on the ride and can do their jobs properly. With these in action, there is no reason why our blood sugar levels would soar up.

And there you have it, yet a few more reasons why ACV is something you should definitely consider, and I must confess that I would be surprised if you are still thinking about whether you should go for it or not. The advantages continue to pour in from various research, and the number of ACV fans is on the rise.

We have read about how ACV maintains blood sugar level and how it helps maintain a healthy heart. Now comes the time to discover how this tasty treat helps us in maintaining our body's pH level. Yes, we discussed it a little earlier as well, but now, we will be getting into the finer details. Oh, and did I mention I will share some celebrity success stories as well? Yes, there is more to come in the next chapter!

Chapter 5:

Alkaline All the Way

Straight away, I am not referring to the alkaline batteries. As useful as they may be, they have no purpose here within this book. I am actually referring to the body's natural state, the alkaline nature that it is supposed to maintain.

They say what is natural can simply not be bested. I genuinely believe that is the case when it comes to our human body. The way our bodies are designed is just a feat far too extraordinary in its own right.

Our body is naturally found in an alkaline state. That means our pH levels go north of number seven, which is the neutral point. Then, there is the paradoxical irony that our stomach holds one of the most potent and corrosive acids on earth, and that too is natural. I can never imagine touching any form of acid, let alone being near an acid that will burn right through the skin. Surely, nature knows how to keep the balance and allow us to lead a healthy life.

With that said, however, some things still end up going wrong for us. There was a time where I thought getting sick was more of a viral thing than anything else. True, but did you know that you can only get sick if your body is no longer in its natural alkaline state?

Dr. Otto H. Warburg, a Nobel Prize winner, discovered that diseases can never form or develop in an alkaline environment, and that includes something as massive as cancer (Natural Food Pantry, 2017). That is quite a statement if you come to think about it. Naturally, it further cements the importance of our alkaline state of the body than ever before. If cancer cannot develop in an alkaline environment, nothing can.

This chapter, then, will look into the significance of the alkaline body, the pH balance, and reflect on what exactly makes the pH balance such an important aspect of our lives. We will also dive into the ACV world and see how ACV, despite being acidic in nature, helps us in maintaining a proper pH balance.

Alkaline 101

By now, we know our body's natural composition shows alkaline nature. There are foods that are rather acidic, and then there are the ones that aren't. The problem is that we have no way of telling the acidity of the food we are eating unless we keep a chart right next to ourselves and use that as a reference. This is not always ideal as you might be dining out with friends or family, and carrying a chart around with you might make you look a little strange.

Instead, I have listed some of the everyday food items and categorized them with their respective pH values. You can note this down somewhere and try to memorize the ones you eat frequently. Having a bit of knowledge is better than having no knowledge at all.

To begin this section, let us first look at these food items and try to see if we can maintain a balanced pH level throughout the day. There is no reason to worry if the results seem to be tilting a little to one side, as we are only trying to identify the situation first. Resolving the situation is our next step, and we shall do that with full knowledge and preparation.

The pH Breakdown

For the benefit of those who may never have read or heard of a pH scale, here is a quick introduction.

- The pH scale goes from 0 to 14.
- Everything in existence falls somewhere within this range.
- The acidic range is from 0 to 6, 0 being the most acidic substance.
- 7 is the neutral zone, which is where we usually find distilled water. It is neither acidic nor alkaline in nature.

- Anything above 7 to 14 is basic or alkaline in nature, 14 being the highest alkaline point.

Eagle-eyed readers may have noticed that I used two terms: basic and alkaline. Books on chemistry, whichever you might pick, define an alkali as a particular type of base. All alkalis are bases, but not all bases are alkalis, as not all of the bases can dissolve in water. While this may not be as important for this book, it is still something that one should know. You never know when you might get into a conversation where one person might be using the word base instead of an alkali. Understanding the difference will ensure that you know exactly what they are referring to.

As for our bodies, the normal pH range is between 7.35 and 7.45, and that means it is neither neutral or acidic. If anything, it is slightly alkaline in nature, emphasis on the word 'slightly' as more often than not, people tend to get it wrong.

Now comes the exciting part. Considering that our body is just north of the neutral zone, it can quickly lose its balance and tip over to one side. This has everything to do with what we eat, what we drink, and our habits, such as smoking. Food items are found within each range described above.

Side note: Food items generally fall on the lower end of the scale (acidic), with only a few managing to go slightly north of the neutral zone.

Grab a pen and some paper, and try to note down all that you ate today. Once done, find where your balance lies and see if you can munch on some of the counterparts to balance your pH levels out.

Highly Acidic Food Items and Drinks

- Sugar - Yes, you read that right!
- Grains
- Some dairy products
- Processed foods, nearly all of them
- Sodas or any other sweetened drink
- Fish
- High-protein foods
- Protein supplements
- Fresh meats
- Processed meats

Fruits and Juices

For this list, keep in mind that the first one is the most acidic, and the last one is the least acidic in nature. Their respective pH values are also provided next to their names.

- Lemon juice (2.00 - 2.60)
- Limes (2.00 - 2.80)
- Blue plums (2.80 - 3.40)
- Grapes (2.90 - 3.82)
- Pomegranates (2.93 - 3.20)
- Grapefruits (3.00 - 3.75)
- Blueberries (3.12 - 3.33)
- Pineapples (3.20 - 4.00)
- Apples (3.30 - 4.00)
- Peaches (3.30 - 4.05)
- Oranges (3.69 - 4.34)
- Tomatoes (4.30 - 4.90)

(Katherine Marengo, 2018)

It is generally a rule of thumb that citrus fruits have a lower pH value. This means they fall on the acidic side of the pH scale. If you have felt ulcer issues or refluxes, it is a signal which denotes that your body is brimming with acidic contents.

Things are pretty much the same when it comes to fruit juices. Why am I highlighting this separately? The reason is a bit more important than you might think. Acid can react with your teeth and gums, making them vulnerable and weak. This is the sole reason why the drinking straw was created. That person allowed us to enjoy every sip of nature's finest without bringing the acidic content in direct contact with our teeth.

To find out if certain fruits are healthy for you to have regularly, test it out and see if it brings about any kind of upper digestive symptoms. If not, that fruit can be consumed on a daily basis.

When it comes to vegetables, you may imagine that all of them are alkaline in nature, right? You might be surprised to know that not all of them are alkaline. Some of these are acidic in nature, and these include some of the most commonly consumed vegetables in existence.

Fresh Vegetables

- Sauerkraut (3.30 - 3.60)
- Cabbage (5.20 - 6.80)
- Beets (5.30 - 6.60)
- Corn (5.90 - 7.50)
- Mushrooms (6.00 - 6.70)

- Broccoli (6.30 - 6.85)
- Collard greens (6.50 - 7.50)

Food with Low-Acid Values

- Soy, soybeans, tofu, tempeh
- Yogurt and milk (unsweetened)
- Most fresh vegetables (including potatoes)
- Mustard
- Nutmeg
- Herbs and spices (not including salt)
- Beans
- Lentils
- Some whole grains, like millet
- Herbal teas
- Olive oil
- Avocados

Consuming any of the above is okay, as long as you are limiting the intake and countering it with plenty of water or any alkaline substances. Tilt the scale far too much to the acidic side, and you risk exposing yourself to problems of the worst kind. These include, but are not limited to, acidity and kidney stone formation. Ask anyone who may have gone through the ordeal of passing a stone, and they will confirm that it is one of the most excruciating pains you can come to know of.

Too much acidity also puts you at risk of cancer, heart issues, and other fatal diseases. This is generally seen in the cases of people who have ridiculously high doses of phosphoric acid. This type of acid is quite commonly used in darker drinks and sodas. Avoid that as much as you can and stick to water or any other healthy drinks.

Lastly, being exposed to a lot of acidic content can lead to bone and muscle deterioration. Calcium, found within the bones, is used by our bodies to naturally balance the pH levels when they get too acidic in nature. If our bones are weak, they will contain less calcium. The less calcium there is, the more we end up losing the battle against acidity.

For those who might be wondering when I will show the alkaline food items, I assure you, most edible items do not go beyond the ranges defined above. Anything above that is a risk to our health if consumed in large quantities. Remember, our bodies are barely north of the neutral zone, and consuming anything containing more than a pH value of 8 would cause us to experience a bitter taste and a very unpleasant feeling.

We consume various kinds of fruits, vegetables, and other food sources every day. That is not out of desire but out of need. Without them, we could not fathom leading a life, let alone a healthy one. It is rather easy to lose track of these figures and end up creating a more acidic environment within our body. Naturally, that opens a doorway to many issues.

Balancing such an issue can be tricky. To begin with, no fruits or vegetables come with these pH numbers on them. Secondly, there is no proper way to find out your current pH standings, either. Fortunately, though, this is exactly where the good old apple cider vinegar comes in to save the day.

ACV, despite being acidic in nature, does play a fantastic role and can help many balance out their body’s pH levels. It is considered one of the most excellent remedies known to man to treat issues like heartburn and other such ailments caused by the imbalance of your body's pH.

The internet is brimming with various theories, answers, and responses. While these theories and suggestions go their own separate ways, one thing is common; ACV does assist in maintaining the body's alkaline nature, despite being acidic itself.

This is made possible by the complex nature of our bodies. Whatever you eat or drink is broken down into soluble and consumable bits and pieces. Whatever is unneeded is then passed out through urination. ACV helps create a soothing effect and stops issues like heartburn, acid reflux, and such problems that are otherwise common.

Another thing to note here is that while vinegar is acidic in nature, apples have contents which are alkaline in nature. The acetic acid does help in digestion, but the apple contents help in allowing your body to recover its alkaline state. It should also be noticed that ACV contains calcium, which, if you recall from earlier, takes the leading charge in stabilizing the pH balance of your body. With the added supply of calcium, our body gets more to work with and hence balances out the pH imbalance that may have been caused due to the consumption of acidic foods and drinks.

There is a reason why ACV is considered one of the most excellent home remedies for heartburn and other digestive issues. The reason is simple: it works like a charm! You always have the option of taking an antacid pill, but when you have a natural way of balancing pH levels, why opt for the pills?

I know quite a few people who prefer to stay on antacids because they apparently work faster and, as per some, have negligible side-effects. I am not too sure if that is the case. The internet certainly doesn't feel the same way either. Using chemicals and pills to resolve heartburn and other digestive issues can lead to some nasty problems. ACV, on the other hand, is always a safer option, provided that it is consumed in a limited quantity.

Apart from these qualities and benefits, there are many other ways it helps us balance our pH levels. We will look into this a little more in the next few chapters and discover how it helps balance our skin's pH level (yes, our skin has a different pH level).

Some Big Names Who Use ACV

I am not going to suggest a list of names here based on any rumors. I will not refer to tales or any such thing. In fact, I will be listing down some of the biggest names in the television industry who have confessed their special love for apple cider vinegar.

Celebrities are role models for a global audience. With millions of followers, it is a given that whatever they try and suggest, the masses will eagerly and voluntarily follow the same. While some celebrities have made an impact in the wrong manner, willingly or unwillingly, there certainly are many who love to share their health secrets with the world.

There are those who talk about how wonderful the keto diet is, and then there are those who talk about the perks of intermittent fasting. Regardless of which celebrity you follow, there is a significant chance your most admired celebrity might already be using the magical elixir that is apple cider vinegar. Without further ado, let us find out just who these celebrities are and what they may have to say about the wonderful and tasty ACV.

Katy Perry

The American icon that Katy Perry has become has left many fans and critics in sheer awe through the magical use of her voice. She has given the world some of the finest hits to grace our ears. Her melodies and her powerful vocals are a match made in heaven.

Behind the glamour, Katy Perry herself admitted that she has been using apple cider vinegar throughout her life. She has her mother to thank for this, and owing to its continuous use, she continues to have glowing skin and health that is always 100%, which is why she has never missed out on a show due to health-related issues.

That is quite an achievement for a celebrity of any caliber. For not having missed a single show and yet retaining immaculate health, I can honestly not think of any other person or personality who can match such a feat. I am sure there are some out there, but no one is as full of energy as Katy Perry.

Scarlett Johansson

For all the Avengers' fans, say hello to the Black Widow. Yes, the downright gorgeous actress who portrayed the role of Natasha Romanov in the MCU is also a huge fan of apple cider vinegar. She has admitted to using apple cider vinegar in her skincare regimen. If you ever wondered what made her skin look so soft and glowing, now you know her secret.

Megan Fox

One of the most desired actresses out there, she has made her presence felt and redefined beauty ever since she appeared in the *Transformers* series. It is of little surprise to find out that she, too, cannot resist the charming effects of apple cider vinegar.

She claimed that apple cider vinegar helps her out by flushing the entire system of any harmful substances and helps her with her premenstrual syndrome (PMS).

Jennifer Aniston

Okay, this is a unique entry. The world remembers her for that incredibly gorgeous hairstyle, her breath-taking beauty, and the quirky and dynamic character she played on *Friends*. She is the epitome of self-care and an ambassador for apple cider vinegar. She showcases all that is good about the entire ACV world every time she is on screen.

She has been seen continually mentioning her love for the benefits of apple cider vinegar. She prefers using the raw form of ACV as opposed to the filtered one. The raw form can be a bit of a challenge to sip unless you add a little honey into the mix. She has not exactly mentioned how she prefers taking it, but she has certainly informed various channels and magazines that she prefers taking it first thing in the morning.

Her perseverance and consistency allowed ACV to fully shine bright and provide her with all the possible health benefits. Despite her age, she looks as young and glowing as ever.

She has mentioned, on various occasions, that ACV has allowed her to enjoy a heap of benefits. Some of the main ones are:

- Improved digestion
- No room for bloating
- Increased energy
- Clearer skin
- A well-balanced body pH

The internet is awash with information regarding Aniston's diet routine, special emphasis being put on the ACV. Her iconic looks, her plentiful energy, and her incredible physique are some of the results of using ACV regularly.

Remember, while ACV itself is quite beneficial, it does take time and consistency before you can fully see the results. Jennifer Aniston has done just that; she managed to stick to it, and the results are now there for the world to see and marvel in.

Gwyneth Paltrow

Some of you might have raised an eyebrow or even Googled to see who this lady is, just to find out that you already know her as Pepper Potts. Yes, the love interest and wife of Tony Stark, better known as Iron Man, is also no stranger to the world of apple cider vinegar.

Apart from her phenomenal acting career, she has written a complete recipe book (*It's All Good Cookbook*), most of which uses and promotes the use of, yes, you guessed it, apple cider vinegar. For a celebrity of her status writing a book that clearly inclines towards the use of ACV, it is quite a statement.

There are numerous other celebrities who either have a sip of ACV in the morning or prefer to use it as a salad dressing for some added taste. Apple cider vinegar is undoubtedly breaking the headlines almost every day, and there is no end in sight.

If I was to sum it all up in one word as to why people use apple cider vinegar, it would be longevity. Why? You just need to think a little to realize that apple cider vinegar is offering so much, and one of those fringe benefits is a digestive system that is as clean as a whistle. The cleaner you are, the longer you live, and that is a fact.

With a balanced pH level, your body will never leave that comfort zone. As a result, it will block off almost every disease and ailment. The burst of extra energy will ensure that you continue doing what you do best, and the improved digestion will allow for a constant supply of nutrients as whatever you eat will be absorbed more efficiently.

In the coming chapter, we will discuss how the apple cider vinegar helps with our skin. When we talk about skin, we usually refer to everything about the skin. This includes the hair as well, so for those who may have wondered if ACV can do something to improve hair, I have got you covered.

The next chapter will also provide some tips and tricks which can help you reap further benefits. You can record these, note them down, or just memorize them, and then try the same to see the results for yourself. With that said, I will see you again in the next chapter.

Chapter 6:

Clear Your Skin

Hopefully, you weren't gone that long. If you were, welcome back. Now that formalities are out of the way, let us focus on the second biggest reason why everyone is searching for apple cider vinegar:

The skin.

Human beings are classified as social animals with larger brains. We are protected by the largest organ in our body, and that is our skin.

Previously, when we were discussing the pH levels of the body, I highlighted that our skin has a different pH level. Unlike our whole body's pH level, which is alkaline, our skin should ideally maintain a slightly acidic pH value. To be a little more precise, a pH level of 5.5 is what you should be aiming for.

Before we jump into this chapter and see what's what, let us first familiarize ourselves with our skin's pH level. This is something important for everyone to know, as this can honestly help us avoid perils and issues of considerable proportion.

Our skin is continuously fighting off all environmental threats, diseases, bacteria, and so on. It is no wonder why our skin is the first to develop some kind of acne, rashes, or other skin-related issues as it loses its pH balance rather quickly. Unlike the whole body's pH level, we cannot change the pH level of our skin immediately. There is also the problem of aging.

You can try all you would like, but there is absolutely no way to avoid aging unless you somehow end up discovering the fountain of youth like Captain Jack Sparrow did. Aging is constant, and it is a continuous process that starts from the day we are born until the day we die.

With aging, our skin undergoes a lot of changes which may not be apparent at first. Over time, our skin grows more and more acidic. The more it loses its naturally acidic composition, the more it is prone to damage. Everything affects our skin, be it air, smoke, water, pollution, UV rays, or whatever you can think of.

The acid mantle of our skin is the protecting layer, which helps us fight various environmental effects every day. When the pH level of the skin changes, the acid mantle is affected and stops working as it usually should. Issues like rosacea, dermatitis, and eczema are most likely to be the result of such a situation.

In normal circumstances, you would rush to your nearest skin specialist or skin-care center and buy some expensive drugs or topical lotions to fix this. I, however, would recommend sticking to one of the at-home skin pH level check kits. These are extremely simple to use and provide you with accurate results. You can find these at most drug stores in your vicinity.

Once you know your skin's pH level, you can then apply appropriate creams or medications to fix this. However, get the wrong product, and you risk developing over-acidic, or extremely under-acidic, skin. Either way, that's bad news.

I will cut to the chase here and address the obvious; this is all too complicated. Buy a pH level check kit, then apply the right kind of product that may cost a fortune or might not even be available. If not, we may end up adding to the problem instead. With that said, however, there is an easy fix to the entire situation: apple cider vinegar.

In the previous chapter, we did see how some celebrities use ACV for skin care, such as Jennifer Aniston. There is little room to doubt the authentic nature of ACV as anything dubious would have cast a grim shadow on ACV's reputation, and celebrities would have never touched something they were unsure of. This should further give us the encouragement we need to try out ACV and see just how effective it can be for glowing, soft, and clear skin. Say goodbye to acne problems and other skin-related issues because ACV is not just a solution for today; it will work for as long as you use it.

Unique Uses for ACV

I will have to be honest here and admit that for me, I was always more drawn to the skin-related benefits that ACV has to offer. However, what came as a bit of a surprise to me was the fact that ACV can be consumed in more ways than just orally.

This changed everything for me, and I am sure the same might have left you with a heightened interest when I initially mentioned how ACV could be applied topically for acne purposes.

Apple cider vinegar has certain properties that truly makes it unique. ACV comes into its own when it is used during the summer. The summertime is usually when our skin faces the sun at its harshest. It can push our skin to develop acne, pimples, suntan, sunburn, sunspots, and so much more. To counter that, let me give you some tips you can use whenever the summer sun shines too brightly upon you and irritates your skin:

For Sunburns

Ouch! Sunburn is never a pleasant thing to encounter. It leaves you with extra-sensitive skin that feels like it is on fire if someone touches it. Fortunately, apple cider vinegar has just the cure. Not only does it help soothe the pain, but it also acts as a catalyst to speed up the healing process.

1. Take four cups of water and mix it with half a cup of ACV.

2. Use a clean cloth and douse it in the mixture.

3. Apply to the affected area.

4. Massage gently for a while.

5. Repeat a few times daily for a few days until the condition improves.

For Acne & Pimples

1. Mix half a teaspoon raw and unfiltered ACV in a bowl of filtered water.

2. Soak a little cotton ball into this particular mixture.

3. Apply on skin.

4. Leave it on for around 10 minutes before washing it off with luke-warm water.

5. Repeat a few times every day.

The results will leave you astonished. Sooner than you might imagine, you will have skin glowing ever so brightly, with softness and beauty that will catch quite some attention.

Why this happens is simple; it is because the apple cider vinegar has antibacterial properties and contains an antifungal substance, which in turn assists our skin and keeps our pores from absorbing damaging elements, such as dust, oil, and bacteria.

ACV for Exfoliation

Yes, ACV can indeed help you with the exfoliation process. Surprised? Don't be. For soft and supple skin, ACV is the perfect recipe. With its alpha hydroxy acid, it dramatically eases the process by removing the dead skin cells and revealing a layer of healthy new ones.

1. In a bathtub of warm water, pour in about two cups of apple cider vinegar.

2. Ease yourself into the bathtub and lie in it for around 15 minutes.

3. Let the acid soak in.

4. For best results, make this a routine practice.

ACV as Skin Toner

Owing to its astringent properties, ACV works like a charm as it helps increase blood flow to the skin and magically reduces the pores. It is an ideal tool for those suffering from oily skin.

1. Mix two tablespoons of ACV with a glass of filtered water. If needed, add a few drops of your favorite essential oil.

2. Use a clean cotton ball and apply the mixture on your face.

3. Leave the mixture on for a few minutes and then rinse it off with cold water.

4. Use this once or twice, at most, every day.

ACV Against Wrinkles

Utilizing the same alpha hydroxy acids, apple cider vinegar is terrific if you wish to have those fine lines and wrinkles disappear. Sure enough, it may not be able to remove all of them. Still, the job it does is far more surprising than you might think.

1. Use a little cotton ball and dab it directly in the ACV, just a few.

2. Apply it directly onto your age spots and wrinkles.

3. Leave it on for around 30 minutes before rinsing it off with cold water.

4. Make this a routine activity, doing it twice a day for six weeks to see improvement.

In Case of Irritation

While ACV is harmless to most people, there have been some rare cases where people have reported elevated irritation when applying ACV topically. If that is the case, rinse with cold water immediately and stop applying ACV directly to your skin. It is also imperative to note that ACV should never come into contact with your eyes. If it does, rinse your eyes with cold water until the pain subsides. If needed, consult a doctor for further action.

Apple cider vinegar is quite versatile to have in your kitchen. Its benefits continue to grow in number and intensity as it is utilized every single day. However, since we are discussing the benefits of ACV for skin, our skin does contain hair as well. I am not referring to the hair we pluck and remove, but the hair that matters.

Apple Cider Vinegar for Hair

We all have various hairstyles, and then we have different hair types. Some of us are graced with silky and straight hair, while others are fortunate enough to have significant volume and strength. Regardless of what your hair type, color, or length is, apple cider vinegar can certainly add some much-needed quality and help us fight off a few major hair-related issues as well.

Our scalp, just like our skin, has its natural pH level. Since apple cider vinegar is rich in acetic acid, it holds quite a lot of benefits for the scalp and the hair in general, and this is good news for us all. With apple cider vinegar in our kitchen, there is no reason why we should continue spending hundreds of dollars on a single hair product that promises to deliver, yet always ends in disappointment.

Apple cider vinegar comes loaded with all the essential components that strengthen our scalp and rid it of all the build-up and deposits that tend to gather, even after thorough washes with shampoo. A little known fact, shampoo can leave deposits on your scalp, and that can eventually lead to all sorts of problems, including hair loss.

This all sounds great, but how do you know if your hair needs an apple cider vinegar treatment? Are there any specific signs to keep an eye out for? As it turns out, yes, there are.

When our hair starts feeling frizzy, brittle, or dull, these symptoms denote that our scalp is turning alkaline in nature. Counter that, and your hair texture and feel will return to normal; you may even feel a significant difference as your hair will now be healthier than ever before.

One of the most significant issues we run into with hair-related problems is that we do not pay much attention to our hair's needs. Just like the engine of a car needs an oil change after a certain number of miles, our hair too needs fuel to survive and remain healthy. Protein is the source that can easily be provided through various hair tonics and oils, but that is only treating the hair itself. ACV treats the scalp like no other and you will see the difference in how healthy your hair will look as you stay consistent with using it.

ACV has picked up quite a few titles, and it might not come as a surprise that it is considered an excellent disinfectant. For minor hair problems, which include itchiness and minor infections, it might help to control the bacteria or the fungi that tend to grow at the top of our scalp. You may be thinking, "Forget the theories, show me how!"

We are going to prepare a simple hair wash consisting of apple cider vinegar. This hair wash will be easy to use and should pose no harm. Take notes, if needed, as this will certainly impress you with the results.

1. Mix water with a couple of tablespoons of ACV.

2. Once you are finished shampooing and conditioning, apply this mixture evenly and work it into your scalp.

3. Let the mixture remain there for a few minutes.

4. Rinse with water.

If you are someone who does not like the strong smell of ACV, feel free to throw in a drop or two of your favorite essential oil to give it a more appealing fragrance. Use this mixture a few times a week. For the mixture, use less than five tablespoons of ACV, as any more might cause issues.

Knowing If ACV Is Right for You

As always, some cases have reported unpleasant sensations or irritation on the scalp. If that is the case, stop using the ACV mixture on your scalp and consult a doctor to have the issue diagnosed. This generally happens if your scalp is already suffering other ailments that the ACV cannot treat.

You can first initiate a test by using a diluted mixture and applying it to a test region. After a few minutes, if you feel a burning sensation or itchiness, it means the ACV mixture is not for you.

Why Should I Try This?

Let's face it, we all live in a world where good looks matter quite a lot. You can have the finest, softest, and most glowing skin, but all your good looks would be spoiled if you have hair that is brittle and frizzy. The same is true if it is the other way around. Maintain both of these, and the world will be noticing you, even if they try not to.

Looking good and feeling good go hand in hand. It is your birthright to look and feel good. Unfortunately, there are far too many issues in the world that consume our time and take our attention. As a result, we tend to overlook the importance of caring for our skin and hair. Eventually, we end up with a weak scalp full of dryness and dandruff, or with skin feeling extra-sensitive to the touch. None of that sounds charming or even remotely pleasant. If that is the case, and you are still not paying attention, you would find yourself running away from crowded places to hide your embarrassment.

Now, you have a way out of this, and it does not cost you a fortune either. All it takes is a bit of commitment and determination. Even if you were to settle for any other chemically created product, you would need to religiously follow a routine before you would see some results. Why waste your energy, money, and time on products that may work for a while but then produce yet another issue, when you can go for a simple ACV recipe and save yourself all that misery?

If you look good, and you know it, your confidence level will rise automatically. You would walk into a crowd, knowing that you will turn heads and attract quite a lot of attention. There may be people whom you can help and be an example to.

Whoever came up with apple cider vinegar either knew its value or was just plain lucky to have come up with such a thing; it has been around for thousands of years, and it continues to impress the world with its virtually limitless uses and benefits.

With apple cider vinegar by your side, you will always feel confident to face pretty much any situation of any magnitude and still come out a winner. You will have all the confidence in the world, backed by various research and celebrities who have vouched for the sheer number of benefits it provides.

Moving forward, we will now look into the chapter that perhaps was your number one reason behind discovering the wonders of apple cider vinegar. We will finally look into how this incredible elixir can help us reduce those extra pounds that have been bothering us for quite some time now. It wouldn't be a complete book if I were to avoid talking about weight loss. "Weight Loss for the Win" is our next chapter, and I shall see you there!

Chapter 7:

Weight Loss for the Win

Weight loss is the most searched keyword of today. Every other person you run into is looking for an effective way to lose weight and shed off those extra pounds somehow. While some might succeed, others are left worrying about their physical appearance.

It is slightly worrying how people go to extremes where they are ready to undergo surgeries, take pills that pose a risk to health, and try out methods that are neither backed by common sense nor scientific studies.

The most "obvious" way to lose weight would be to starve yourself to a near-death experience, but is that necessary? What is the point in doing something that will take away the weight but leave you with hundreds of other problems to face? By not eating or by opting for slightly weird diet styles, you are barring your body from gaining energy. Without energy, neither you nor your body would be able to carry out simple tasks that would otherwise not make you break a sweat.

Then, some continue to worry about their 'excessive' weight, which barely tips the scale 5 to 10 pounds at most, and yet they are pulling their hair out as if it is the end of the world. It is good that people care about their weight, but it is pointless to continue worrying about it and not do anything to fix it. We, as human beings, have become experts at thinking we will do something, only to wake up the next day and repeat the same cycle all over again. Until you find that will to break this cycle and do something about it, you will never lose those additional pounds.

Before we go ahead, I need you to promise yourself that you will read and act on whatever you have understood, and not just read and forget. We read tons of material online every day. We even mark some of these as essential and save them on notes and browsers. The next day, we tend to forget, and move on. If that is what you will end up doing, now is the time to turn around and walk away, and I do not wish for you to do that.

You are not alone in this. The Center for Disease Control and Prevention published an alarming figure. Between 2015-2016, almost 40% of adults within the United States were classified as obese (Bubnis, 2020). That figure will have gone up significantly by now.

Obesity is gaining weight beyond control, and that spells disaster from every angle. Obesity is when a person has put on a critically high amount of fat and, as a result, is predisposed to numerous health issues.

Whether you are aiming to lose weight because of health concerns or to look better, I assure you that it is the right move. Losing weight will ensure that you protect you and your body from any further harm. Obesity is associated with a range of diseases and ailments, all of which can attack you at any given time. Besides, being obese already causes you to have balance issues, joint pain, and backaches.

Some of the diseases associated with obesity are:

- Heart diseases
- Stroke
- High blood pressure
- Cancer
- Gallstones and gallbladder issues
- Osteoarthritis
- Gout
- Breathing issues (sleep apnea) and asthma

If that doesn't sound alarming, here is another one for you: An obese person is twice as likely to die well before the national average age compared to a person of healthy weight.

I am not making any of this up to promote the use of ACV. These are official statistics present on various sources. It is indeed a point to worry, a moment to stop and rethink things. The way this rate is creeping up, I would not be surprised if very soon we all learn we are too late to avoid the inevitable.

Nothing in life lies beyond our reach, as all it takes is a bit of will and determination to see us through. We discovered planets and stars billions of miles away because we tried. We learned about so many diseases and found cures and treatments because we tried. Similarly, we can avoid the consequences here as well, only if we genuinely try. And the good news is, we are already halfway through.

To keep the momentum going, let us now dive into our final sections; yes, these are the ones you are most interested in. Let us learn if apple cider vinegar truly is the kind of elixir celebrities and studies claim it to be. Remember, I do not guarantee that everyone will experience the same results. It entirely depends on your body chemistry, any prior ailment or disease, your physical routine, and your consistency. However, it has a very high success rate, and that means you are most likely the kind of person who would experience the benefits of ACV firsthand.

Understanding Weight and Weight Loss

For quite some time now, I have observed a fair number of skeptics out there who continue to question the very nature and benefits of apple cider vinegar, and rightly so.

As human beings, we have every right to understand what exactly we are signing up for, how it will react with our bodies, and what will be the potential outcome of the whole deal. Without having reliable answers to these questions, we simply cannot move any further.

Even if you are a person who wishes to buy a Ferrari or a Lamborghini, you would walk into a showroom and ask a few questions to acquire further information and a sense of satisfaction that your purchase is the right one.

In a very similar manner, I do not discourage you from asking questions, but I would honestly prefer it if people started asking the right questions. For example, I know a person who recently asked me if ACV can help them be better in bed. To be honest, I have no idea as there is no profound research linking performance with ACV. However, had the person asked what else they would need apart from ACV, which could help them up their game, I would have certainly pointed out a healthy exercise routine.

Apple cider vinegar has its limits. Let this part soak in for a minute. We tend to get so excited that we start setting unrealistic goals and expectations. The only way that will end is with a massive disappointment.

However, whatever the limits of ACV may be, I genuinely believe they are more than enough for us to be able to utilize and draw the results we are looking for. With over thousands of studies, there are so many indications which point out that ACV truly can help you with your weight loss goals. But do hold your horses here! To fully understand how this is done, we first need to visit the source and learn why we end up putting on the extra weight. This is necessary to ensure that you do not end up in a vicious cycle where you use ACV to lose weight but continue certain habits that cancel out the effects of the ACV. Makes sense, right? Well then, let's begin.

Every organization in the world that has to do with health will most likely point to the reasons below as the real source of your weight issues. Understand them, recognize them, and then learn how to correct them with a holistic approach and a bit of ACV.

Just Being Lazy

Eating too much never pushes your body to gain weight, no sir! It is our own laziness after consuming so many calories that makes the entire situation worse for us. After eating, our body quite literally pushes more blood and uses the energy to digest the food and break it down for nutrients and other vital resources. After having a belly full, we do not do anything to boost our digestion and provide our body with a reason to burn more calories. The unburnt calories are the source of the problem.

Start exercising or just walking for a while around the house, around the corner, around the block, or wherever you can. By walking, you are burning away the excess calories while the body is busy consuming only the calories it needs. The point to understand here is that our body will never digest more calories or energy than it needs. Whatever is in excess, our body will either flush it out or store it elsewhere for future use.

Make a habit of walking for 15 to 30 minutes after your meals to burn those excess calories off. I will discuss how ACV jumps in a little later, though I have every reason to believe that you already know where this might be going (if so, great!).

"But I do exercise after I eat, yet I am still putting on weight. What gives?" The human body can put on weight even if you exercise regularly. Being lazy is the biggest reason, but there are other underlying causes and symptoms that might promote weight gain.

Diabetic Treatments

It is no secret that diabetic patients do tend to put on quite a lot of weight, especially during their treatments. This is a known side-effect of the insulin people take to help them further manage their blood sugar levels.

You may also have heard of a condition called *hypoglycemia.* It is a condition where a person with diabetes, usually a longstanding case, eats more than needed to prevent low sugar levels. Either way, this can dramatically lead to weight gain.

Another issue found within a diabetic patient is the constant appetite for snacks. This, too, leads to an increased number of calories within the body, more than your body can process and burn. The result is then visible.

Aging

With age comes a big belly; I am sorry, but that is how things are. It has little to do with the number reflecting your years on this earth and more to do with the fact that with this increasing number, our bodies lose the capacity to work more.

There comes a time when even the simplest tasks, such as going up a single flight of stairs, might leave you breathless. That is generally because our internal organs start losing their capacity and function. They erode with time and are no longer as efficient as they used to be. The result would see us troubled with regular tasks. This is precisely the reason why the elderly need assistance to walk, climb stairs, sit, get up, and sleep.

The muscles we have today may no longer be there in a few years. This can be prevented by regularly exercising to ensure that these muscles are always in use. The more inactive a tissue remains, the more it is twice as likely to lose its function entirely as opposed to the ones we continue to use.

With a body that is depreciating, muscles that are fading away will no longer require energy. The less energy your body needs, the less your digestive system will work to break down food into other nutrient forms. This will then leave us with extra calories that once were easily consumed but are no longer required now. See how things are connected here? Exercise is honestly a life-saver.

Steroid Treatments

For people suffering from issues like *Polymyalgia Rheumatica* (PMR), or other matters where steroids are the only treatment, I am afraid I have some bad news. Steroids come packed with numerous side-effects, and weight gain is one of them.

Steroids work in a certain way, and I honestly do not wish to get into the finer details here as that would require chapter after chapter. These are generally prescribed when your immune system fails to work on its own. This synthetic measure that we adopt to help our body deal with issues alters the way our body works. The steroid drug typically alters our body's electrolyte balance, as well as its water balance. It also changes our metabolism. This results in three possible scenarios:

- An increased appetite
- Fluid retention

- Change of location where the body stores fats

The body will start depositing fats in unusual places like the neck, face, or abdomen. Because of the fat redistribution, you are bound to look more plump than you might actually be.

Depending on the dose and the duration of said dose, the weight gain might change from person to person. There are no fixed numbers, but over 70% of the people who have been prescribed steroid drugs report weight gain as a side-effect (Christiano, 2018).

Consult a doctor to look for a possible way out to reduce the weight gain, if not altogether avoid it. While ACV will work, it might not be best in some instances. It is always advisable to consult a doctor if you are a patient of an active disease to ensure that the ACV will not react negatively with your body and prescribed drugs.

Underactive Thyroid

Yet another common issue that many of us are simply unaware of. The state of an underactive thyroid is generally termed as *hypothyroidism.* The thyroid is a gland that produces hormones.

For anyone who may be suffering from hypothyroidism, the thyroid will not produce enough hormones. This then slows the body's metabolism, and we all know what a slowed metabolism can do — it leads to weight gain.

This condition is typically found in older women, but it can still manifest in either sex and at any age. Consult a doctor to find out if you have an underactive thyroid.

Cushing's Syndrome

This is one of those rare conditions, which means you should probably not be worried. However, it is good to have an idea of what this is and how you can spot it in the future. It is generally caused when your body is quite literally brimming with the cortisol hormones.

It can develop in patients who have a long-term steroid treatment underway or who may have a tumor. Once again, it is best to consult a doctor to know the extent of damage fully and take evasive action before it is too late.

Stress

For all who may have heard that stress can lead to increased weight, it is true! There is a catch, though, not everyone might experience the same result.

Our body and mind have unique ways to respond to stressful situations, anxiety, and even depressive moods. Some of us may know how to manage stress levels, while others have a ridiculously hard time dealing with issues. Either way, there is a good chance that you might experience weight gain as a result. On a side note, some lose weight due to stress, but still, it is just as bad!

When people are stressed, they can easily be drawn to eat more. This is a coping mechanism quite a lot of us have. Whenever we feel stressed, we take refuge by eating more than usual. Weight gain from depression, however, can have a profound effect, and not in the right way. It will make you feel more depressed than ever before. This is why there are so many specialists out there, continually trying to remind you to step out of depression and work on your own body and mind. The benefits outweigh the drawbacks of stress and depression any given day.

To manage stress, here are some ways which can significantly help you do just that:

- Exercise
- Pick up a creative hobby
- Talk to a friend/partner
- Walk
- Take a relaxing bath
- Learn breathing exercises

All of these work exceptionally well and can significantly improve your mood and bring your stress levels down almost immediately. Don't take my word for it, try it yourself and find out just how easy it is to manage stress and how wonderful it feels once your weight is managed.

Tiredness

While there is the entire thing of how sleeping more might cause you some harm, it might be a bit surprising to some that sleeping less is even more problematic. To begin with, your mind suffers the most. You lose focus, you cannot regain the energy you need to deal with everyday chores, and then there is the weight gain.

Some studies have theorized that those who sleep less are more likely to gain weight than the ones who may be sleeping a little more. Again, this is just a hypothesis, and it needs further research, but it is still a significant trend.

Fluid Retention

For those who may not know what I am on about, fluid retention is when your body holds onto liquids longer than needed. This, in turn, causes your body parts to swell. Two of the most common examples are:

- Standing for a long duration of time

- Being premenstrual

You may have seen diabetic patients with swollen ankles, and that is precisely how this goes as well. Your body retains fluids more than it needs to, and hence becomes swollen. The more fluids your body retains, the graver the outcome. If you feel shortness of breath, be sure to call an ambulance right away.

Although being swollen isn't exactly gaining weight, then again, you might not realize whether you are putting on weight or retaining fluids. A quick check with the doctor would always serve you well.

Polycystic Ovary Syndrome

And finally, we have PCOS. It sounds horrible, but it is relatively common. It affects how a woman's ovaries work. You may even have already felt some symptoms, such as irregular periods, growing excess hair, finding it hard to get pregnant, and weight gain.

The troubling issue is that we still do not know exactly what causes this condition. However, still, a check with your doctor would provide you with some details that might help your case.

Now we can discuss how to counter weight gain that might have something to do with these commonly reported issues. We already know that exercise is a great way to proceed. Adding ACV to the mix will only amplify the overall results. I did mention a few times that ACV alone cannot do much, and hence you need to seek other methods to couple with the apple cider vinegar. Hopefully, after reading this, you should already have the perfect combination in mind. Exercise and ACV go hand-in-hand and thus should be your ideal choice.

How ACV Helps In Losing Weight

In all the conditions above, or even for those which I may not have mentioned, weight loss is possible. There is no denying that. Now, the only thing we are left with is a challenge: To crack the code and unlock the potential of apple cider vinegar.

Throughout this book, I spoke on various topics, such as holistic living, and whatever I spoke of can truly benefit you. These are the core components you need to fully enjoy the complete array of benefits apple cider vinegar has to offer.

There are various ways you can reduce weight, but I am not willing to end just with a statement. I am aiming to provide you with complete details on how exactly ACV helps you lose weight.

Increased Metabolism

First things first, the most significant element within our body that controls how much weight we gain and how much we lose is our metabolism. If it is slow, our bellies would pop out like jelly. If it is fast, we would be burning through that fat like never before. Naturally, though, it should be right in the middle. As good as that might be for a healthy person, we want to upset the balance and deliberately tilt it for our benefit. It sounds like cheating, but then again, it is what it is.

The vital thing to know here is that apple cider vinegar is known to have a profound impact on metabolic rate. It is homemade, natural, and cost-effective, and that makes it even better than most so-called weight loss solutions. While others might pose some severe side-effects, apple cider vinegar edges them out by minimizing them, if not completely removing them.

Some eat to live, and then some live to eat. While both are fine, the latter does pose some issues. Those who love to eat and munch away on their favorite snacks now and then tend to gain more weight. The only way to avoid that from happening would be to suppress your appetite through the use of pills and drugs. By consuming apple cider vinegar, you effectively suppress your appetite naturally, hence taking away the biggest problem of the lot.

By reducing the appetite, you provide fewer calories for energy, causing your metabolism to increase. Now, your metabolism burns through those calories more effectively, hence consuming all that is good and not storing any excessive calories within the body. The result is you won't grow a belly or gain excess weight.

As an added advantage, your body's pH level will alkalize. This, in turn, helps in the entire weight loss process.

In a glass of water, mix one or two teaspoons of ACV, and drink it before a meal once a day. If you are not a fan of making your own ACV at home, buy one that is high in quality, organic, raw, and unfiltered. You should be able to see the results in about two to four weeks, depending on multiple factors such as your body's chemistry and age.

Decreases Blood Triglycerides

Do not be alarmed by the intimidating name. This is nothing more than a type of fat found within our blood. The body converts all the calories you may not immediately need into triglycerides. The triglycerides are then stored within the fat cells and used as a source of energy between meals.

While this all sounds normal, it can get out of control if you eat a lot. As a result, your body will have far more triglycerides than needed, increasing your risk of suffering a heart attack or stroke.

The leading causes behind an elevated level of triglycerides are smoking, lack of physical exercise, drinking, and some other lifestyle choices such as excessive eating. The worst part is that there are no specific symptoms that can let people know when their triglycerides are high in number. Keeping them under control is quite essential.

Apple cider vinegar helps by bringing these under control just as it would bring your blood sugar level down. There are further studies underway to understand how ACV manages to do that entirely. Whatever the findings may be, we are interested in the result, and that part is already known to be helpful.

Countless Goodness

Do you know how important potassium is for your body? It plays a very significant role in balancing the fluids, muscle contractions, and all the nerve signals.

Apple cider vinegar is an excellent way to ensure a healthy balance as it is effortless to consume food and other items, which may increase the potassium level within the body. It contains 73mg of potassium, roughly around two percent, for every 100 grams. However, care must be taken when consuming ACV while using insulin or any other medicines as there have been reports which claim that certain drugs interact with ACV.

Another benefit you can get out of ACV is that it helps in maintaining a healthy sodium level within the body. Once again, higher sodium levels within the body can lead to quite a lot of complications, and ACV, being acidic, ensures that you never face that situation.

While quite a lot of people consume salt in pretty much everything these days, it should be understood that salt is not exactly healthy to have in your diet. You can face issues like swollen hands or feet, and these are just short-term symptoms. Longer durations can lead to high blood pressure, kidney disease, congestive heart failure, and strokes.

Limiting your intake of salt is necessary, and ACV is a quick way to ensure your body's sodium level is brought back to normal. Once again, care must be taken if you are on medication. Consult a doctor to ensure that ACV will not interact or react with your medicines as it could amplify side effects.

Yet another benefit that follows and helps in weight loss is ACV's incredible ability to improve iron release from the food you consume. Given its acidic nature, it promotes the release of iron from all food sources and thus allows it to be used within the body. The presence of iron is a vital component of our hemoglobin and myoglobin.

Both of these carry oxygen to the cells throughout our bodies. We all know that oxygen is vital to burn anything; as it serves as fuel for fire, it also plays the same role in burning calories. If our body can burn through calories effectively, it can significantly contribute to weight loss, and apple cider vinegar ensures just that.

Here is a more straightforward way of putting this:

ACV leads to the release of iron. → Iron absorption leads to an effective oxygen utilization. → Better oxygen utilization ensures energy consumption. → Energy consumption leads to weight loss.

If you are someone who has been suffering from a lack of sleep or insomnia, you might already know that lack of sleep also contributes to gaining weight. Well, I have some good news for you as well. The magical apple cider vinegar also makes sure that you get a goodnight's sleep, meaning your body receives the time it needs to fix all the problems and deal with all that might otherwise cause you to put on weight.

It is already apparent that apple cider vinegar is more than just a culinary delight. With such an array of advantages, it should not surprise you to know that people use ACV to help them get some much-needed sleep.

A teaspoon of ACV in a warm cup of water with some honey is the way to go. Not only do you get a goodnight's sleep, but you can also wave your sleep issues goodbye. A good sleeping pattern promotes weight loss and ensures you don't have time to grab a few late-night snacks, which are a factor in weight gain.

People who do tend to stay up late have a greater tendency to eat more than usual. The extra calories which find their way inside your body add to the ones already present. The result then should be of no surprise either; your body gains more weight quickly. Through this effective method, you can be sure that you sleep comfortably and peacefully, thus ensuring you do not stay up late, munching on your favorite snacks or whatever you can find in the fridge.

Finally, the problem of eating and yet feeling unsatisfied: It is quite a collective experience for most of us. We tend to eat as much as we want, and however, it never seems to satisfy our hunger. We do not feel as full as we would have hoped for. This keeps the door open for some new food, and we are rather quick to utilize the opportunity to eat that delicious looking pie or dig into the cake we baked yesterday.

Apple cider vinegar ensures that you continue to feel full for a longer duration of time. By doing so, you will automatically avoid any food as your belly would not be craving any of those additional treats. Ever remember eating so much that you felt like you would throw up if you saw more food? It is pretty much like that. Not only would you prefer not to eat, but the mere sight might also cause you to leave the room and take a walk to digest your last meal.

Studies are still underway to discover the potential of this incredible culinary item fully. But do not let that stop you from enjoying the benefits that have already been proven and reported for well over thousands of years. If this were as bad as some claim, apple cider vinegar would have indeed vanished a long time ago. Yet it continues to be the choice of celebrities, athletes, and hundreds of thousands of people around the world.

That further reassures us that there is indeed something that continues to attract attention and provide results that leave others stunned.

In the final chapter of the book, I will be discussing ten incredible recipes I know you will love and find useful. Whether you are looking for weight loss or just jumping into the world of apple cider vinegar because a celebrity you dearly love does the same thing, these recipes are sure to give you the start you need to experience the best.

Hopefully, any doubts you may have had when you started this book have been dealt with, and I honestly hope that you have found the answer you were looking for. Reading is only half the fun, though; it is time to taste the remainder and experience the results for yourself.

Chapter 8:

Recipes for Success

Wow! The journey thus far has been full of facts and addressed quite a lot of issues and myths that have circulated ever since I can remember. I have given it my best to ensure all questions posed by the masses got a justified answer.

We have seen in detail all the aspects related to this wonderful invention; all but one, the recipes that involve ACV as the core ingredient. Of course, we knew we would bump into those sooner or later, right?

In this final chapter, we will be looking at some effortless and equally incredible recipes that are sure to leave your taste buds tingling. What's more, you will be heading forward in achieving your targets, whatever they may be, through the use of these recipes revolving around the use of ACV.

We will be looking at various recipes that will cover essential things, like the morning tea to the ones you can rely on for a good night's sleep. All of these recipes are easy and should pose no issues, even if you are someone who has never set foot in the kitchen.

Apple cider vinegar is all about healthy living, but I highly recommend that you not rely exclusively on ACV. Pick up some complementing routines or habits such as regular exercise, improved diet, or a holistic way of living. Whatever you choose, apple cider vinegar will ensure that the results are achieved faster, without compromising the quality or jeopardizing your health. With that said, let us start preparing some incredible recipes and finally taste them.

The Recipes

Throughout this chapter, you will be provided with recipes you will come to know and love, leaving you with a pleasant taste and all the benefits you have read so far. I assure you, you will not be missing out on any of the advantages, nor will any of the apple cider vinegar's goodness be taken away from you.

While there are hundreds of recipes out there, we will only be focusing on easy-to-make and useful recipes. The ones that involve cooking typically consume more time and effort. Apart from the recipes covered in this book, there are numerous resources available online you can look through to find additional delicious recipes to try out for yourself. Feel free to search for these if you wish to kick things up a notch.

Beverages with ACV

Limeade ACV Drink

Who doesn't like a good limeade? While apple cider vinegar is great on its own, it can be a bit of a challenge to adjust to the strong taste it has. This is why I would recommend giving this recipe a try instead. It is a must-have for people who love citrusy drinks.

To make your very own limeade apple cider vinegar drink, all you need is:

- One and a half tablespoon of apple cider vinegar
- One tablespoon of fresh lime juice
- One teaspoon of Stevia (or any other organic sweetener, such as honey)
- Two cups of cold water

I did say the recipes were simple, right? Simply mix these, and that's it! To make the most of the drink, serve it cold.

The taste is sure to leave you with a jolt of energy, as well as the goodness of both the lime juice and the apple cider vinegar.

Ginger Spice ACV Drink

Have an upset tummy? Or perhaps you just like that spicy kick of the ginger. Regardless, this drink is sure to surprise you with an astonishingly exquisite taste. It is also quite useful if you do have an upset stomach, as it can significantly ease your pains and provide you much-needed relief.

To prepare this one, all you need is:

- One tablespoon of apple cider vinegar
- ¼ teaspoon of ground ginger
- One teaspoon of Stevia (or any other sweetener of your choice)
- Two cups of cold water

Mix these, and you have a drink that not only tastes good but also does good for your belly.

Apple Pie ACV Drink

Apple pie is simply the finest delight I can think of. The flavor is delicious, provided that it is made right. So, how can we infuse the great taste of apple pie with apple cider vinegar?

The way to do so is rather straightforward, but the taste you get once you do it right is far better than you may imagine. To create this unique drink, all you need is:

- One tablespoon of apple cider vinegar
- Two tablespoons of organic apple juice
- ¾ teaspoon of your favorite sweetener
- ¼ teaspoon of ground cinnamon
- Two cups of cold water

The added cinnamon adds a kick to the drink, giving it a burst of flavor and a refreshing fragrance. Serve this to any guests as well and be ready to have a bit of a fanbase. This one is extra sweet, and that makes it a worthy addition to have right after a good dinner.

Honey-Cayenne ACV Drink

This drink is an ideal way to go for those who do not mind having a bit of natural sugar involved. Since cayenne is known to jump-start your metabolism, you will certainly feel the effects, and that is just an added advantage apart from its great taste.

Unlike the other drinks, however, I do recommend that you use warm water for this one. This is to ensure that the honey dissolves properly. Once the drink is ready, you can either have it warm or pop it in the fridge and serve chilled. This is also a great remedy for soothing your throat, if sore.

To make this drink, you need:

- One tablespoon of apple cider vinegar
- Two tablespoons of honey (preferably raw and local)
- One dash of cayenne pepper
- Two cups of warm or hot water

Mix the ingredients. Serve at the temperature you please and let the magic of this drink take over.

Fizzy ACV Drink

Okay, I confess I am not great at naming recipes. However, since there are many variations to this recipe, I leave it up to you to decide what to call it.

This recipe is perhaps the simplest of the lot. It only takes three ingredients and is ready to be served in under two minutes.

To make this, you need:

- One tablespoon of apple cider vinegar
- One tablespoon of lemon juice (organic, not from concentrate)
- One and a half cups of soda water of your choice

Mix these and enjoy its refreshing taste.

Apple Cider Vinegar Morning Tea

If you are like me and prefer a good cup of tea in the morning to kick-start the day, you are certainly going to love this one. Not only do you get the much-needed energy flowing within your body, but it is also a great drink if you are looking for some proper old-fashioned detoxification.

For a good serving for one, you will need:

- One cup of warm or hot water
- Two tablespoons of apple cider vinegar
- Two tablespoons of lemon juice
- One tablespoon of honey
- One teaspoon of cinnamon
- One dash of cayenne

Mix these and stir well. The resulting tea will soon be your source of renewed energy and freshness. It tastes good and is equally useful for your health as well.

Apple Cider Vinegar Cocktail

Everyone enjoys a good cocktail, and this should be a drink to go for right before your meals. I prefer mine before dinner, but you can use it when you want.

The drink combines the rich tastes of organic raw honey and apple cider vinegar, infusing them to make one smooth cocktail.

For this, you only need three things:

- One cup of warm water
- One tablespoon of organic raw honey
- One tablespoon of apple cider vinegar

Mix these ingredients and let the honey dissolve. If you are using cold water, it may take a little longer. When ready, serve chilled for the best taste.

Apple Cider Vinegar Detox for Workouts

While this drink can either be taken before or after a workout, I prefer mine after a workout. Once again, I leave it up to you to decide how you would prefer yours.

This drink is quite similar to the ones already mentioned above, but it is mighty effective. To make this quick detox drink, you will need:

- One cup of water (warm or cold)
- One tablespoon of honey
- One tablespoon of apple cider vinegar

- Fresh lime juice
- Optional: salt to taste

I prefer the drink with a hint of salt, but if you are not too happy with the idea of combining salt with this recipe, you can omit that. Mix these, and your detox drink before or after a workout is ready to go.

This drink is something that will go a long way in helping you regain the energy lost after a workout. It helps restore quite a lot of energy in your body, allowing you to cope with any sudden physical demands.

Fire Cider

Do not be intimidated by the name. This is one incredible health tonic to have in your fridge. It is a terrific immune booster and provides layers of taste for those who prefer quality drinks.

Do note that this recipe does take some time; four weeks to be precise!

This is a combination of quite a few elements in play, giving it that incomparable taste. To create this one, you will need:

- Half cup of ginger root (peeled freshly and grated)
- Half cup of horseradish root (freshly grated)

- One medium onion (chopped)
- Ten cloves of garlic (Either crushed or chopped)
- Two jalapeno peppers (organic and chopped)
- One lemon, juice and zest
- Two tablespoons of dried rosemary leaves
- One tablespoon of turmeric powder
- ¼ teaspoon cayenne pepper
- Three to four cups of apple cider vinegar
- ¼ cup of organic and raw honey

Wow, that is quite a lot. Now, here is a step-by-step guide to ensure you get this drink set up and running so you can taste it for yourself.

1. In a quart-sized glass jar, add the ginger, onion, garlic, horseradish, jalapeno peppers, rosemary, cayenne powder, turmeric, and lemon zest and juice.

2. Fill up the jar with apple cider vinegar until it reaches the top of the jar. At this point, all the ingredients should be covered or submerged to prevent any spoilage.

3. Use a piece of natural parchment paper to cover the lid. This is to ensure that the apple cider vinegar does not touch the metal lid. If you have a plastic lid, use that instead.

4. Shake the jar well and store it in a cool and dark place for a period of 4 weeks.

5. Just like with the ACV, shake the jar now and then to ensure the contents are active.

6. After a month, use a strainer or your good old cheesecloth to strain all the solids out. Extract as much liquid as you can into a clean jar. You can use the solids for stir-fry, or simply discard them if you would like.

7. Add honey to the reserved liquid and continue to stir until incorporated.

8. Taste the liquid and add additional honey if needed.

9. Seal in a container and store it in the refrigerator.

10. Drink one or two tablespoons when needed.

This drink is packed with taste and has quite a punch. Let guests and friends try it out as well, and be sure to provide them the recipe because, so far, everyone I know has asked for mine!

Ginger Switchel

I love the way this one sounds, but I love the taste even more. It is an excellent combination of flavors and packs in some genuinely healthy goodness.

To create this, all you need is:

- Two tablespoons of apple cider vinegar
- Four teaspoons of your favorite sweetener
- ¼ teaspoon of ground ginger
- One cup of hot water

Mix these up nicely and let them cool down in a refrigerator for two hours. Don't forget to strain the ginger using a fine sieve or cheesecloth. Before serving, shake the contents and enjoy. For an extra hit of taste, add some sparkling water with ice.

There you have it then—10 incredibly flavorful drinks to keep you going forward. Now, we shall turn over to the other side which involves a bit of cooking. Gear up and grab your notepad as some of these may need a little practice and time to perfect.

Meals with ACV

If you thought you could only create drinks using ACV, let me be the first one to surprise you with a new fact:

you can cook with ACV as well. Yes, these taste incredible; and yes, they offer all the goodness you generally would get in the drinks I mentioned in the previous section.

Put on your chef's hat, lay out your tools, and let's get cooking. This is going to be fun and rewarding.

Grilled Cheese Sandwich with Tomato Chutney

Whenever I hear the word 'chutney,' I cannot help but say, "Yummy!" If you are someone who relates to this passion for chutneys as I do, or if you are someone who has never had the chance to try out a chutney before, this is a perfect way to start.

For this recipe, you will need:

- Tomato Chutney
    - One tablespoon of pickling spice (your choice of the mixture)
    - One tablespoon of olive oil
    - One large shallot, finely chopped
    - ½ cup of apple cider vinegar
    - Two tablespoons of brown sugar
    - ½ teaspoon of salt

    - One and a quarter pounds of chopped tomatoes
    - ½ cup of golden raisins
- Whole grain bread
- Slices of cheese
- Butter

In my case, for the pickling spice mixture, I used cloves, cinnamon, ginger, mustard seeds, bay leaves, dill seeds, black pepper, chili, allspice, and coriander. You can use whatever combination that suits your taste.

Let us look at the chutney first:

1. In a cheesecloth, tie in all the pickling spices and set aside.

2. In a deep and non-reactive saucepan, heat olive oil on medium heat. Add the shallots and sauté them until they are translucent.

3. Add the remaining ingredients to the saucepan and bring them to a boil.

4. After reaching a boil, reduce the heat and simmer without cover.

5. Stir occasionally for 20 minutes. Adjust the taste by adding vinegar, salt, or sugar.

6. Simmer and stir for another 30 minutes, until the mixture is thick.

7. Remove from heat and let it cool down completely.

8. Remove and discard the pickling spices.

9. Store the chutney in a container and refrigerate.

The chutney has a long shelf life, so you can keep it refrigerated for around a month. Now for the final step:

1. Butter up both sides of the whole grain bread.

2. Add slices of your favorite cheese.

3. Add as much chutney as you prefer and spread evenly. For best results, add layers of cheese slices and chutney.

4. Grill on a hot pan until crispy. Enjoy!

Chickpea Waldorf Salad

Whenever we talk about healthy living and eating, salads automatically come to mind. It should be of no surprise then that this entry has made its way here.

Delicious, tasty, and healthy, this recipe is sure to provide you with a salad you will come to love.

To cook for serving four, you will need:

- Half a cup of full-fat yogurt
- Two tablespoons of apple cider vinegar
- One teaspoon of Dijon mustard
- One teaspoon of honey
- Half teaspoon of fine sea salt
- Half teaspoon of crushed red pepper flakes
- ¼ teaspoon of freshly ground black pepper
- One can of chickpeas, thoroughly drained and rinsed
- Two ribs of celery, finely chopped
- One medium apple, chopped into chunks
- One cup of red grapes
- ½ cup of diced red onions
- ¼ cup of chopped parsley
- ½ cup of walnuts, roughly chopped
- Four cups of fresh spinach

Now for the step-by-step guide to this exquisite salad:

1. Make the yogurt dressing by mixing yogurt, mustard, apple cider vinegar, salt, honey, pepper, and crushed red pepper flakes in a bowl. Mix them until well combined.

2. In a separate large bowl, add the chickpeas, apple, grapes, celery, onions, walnuts, and parsley. Add in the dressing and toss until it is evenly distributed. Refrigerate the salad for around 30 minutes before serving.

3. Serve on fresh spinach.

Colorful, tasty, and healthy; all three boxes ticked correctly.

Creamy Vegan Queso Dip

If you are a vegan and you love a good queso dip, I have just the recipe for you. For the final recipe, we will be looking at one of my all-time favorite recipes.

It is easy to make and tastes great. I have served this to guests and have received incredible feedback, which further assures me this is a recipe that truly lives up to the reputation.

To make this one, you will need:

- Two tablespoons of olive oil

- Half a large yellow onion, finely diced

- Three cloves of garlic, minced
- Two large carrots, finely chopped
- One cup of thinly sliced butternut squash
- Two teaspoons of kosher salt, divided
- One teaspoon of ground cumin
- ½ teaspoon of chili powder
- ¼ teaspoon of freshly ground black pepper
- One cup of low-sodium vegetable broth
- One can (four ounces) of green chilies, drained
- One and a half cups of unsweetened, plain almond milk
- One cup of raw cashew, soaked for 30 minutes and drained
- ¼ cup of nutritional yeast
- ½ cup of chunky tomato salsa
- One tablespoon of apple cider vinegar

Time to look at the step-by-step guide to cook this one:

1. In a large saucepan, heat the olive oil on medium heat.

2. Add the onions and garlic, and sauté until they are soft.

3. Add in the butternut squash, carrots, a teaspoon of salt, chili powder, cumin, and black pepper.

4. Cook, and occasionally stir every couple of minutes.

5. Add in the vegetable broth and simmer until the vegetables are soft and tender. They should be soft enough to be smoothly blended in a blender.

6. Transfer the contents into a blender. Add in the green chilies, almond milk, yeast, salsa, cashews, ACV, and the remaining salt.

7. Blend until the mixture reaches a thick, creamy consistency.

8. Gently heat the mixture in a saucepan to bring up the temperature before serving with tortilla chips. Garnish with your favorite topping.

This recipe will typically provide you with four cups, which is good for around 16 servings. It is ideal for a larger group, and it can be stored in the fridge for up to five days.

This then wraps up all the recipes I have thoroughly enjoyed and wanted to share with the rest of the world. This also brings the final chapter to a conclusion.

Conclusion

Apple cider vinegar has been hailed as one of the finest home-made remedies on Earth. Whoever came up with this recipe might be looking down on us today and thinking, "Wow, I never thought this could be such a massive thing!"

The wonders of the great ACV continue to astonish the world. Every passing day, a new recipe for success comes along, or another research paper gets published that claims just how healthy and beneficial apple cider vinegar is.

In all the excitement, it is easy to fall for the wrong information and end up harming yourself. This is why I decided to put together all the information and ideas I know of that truly define what apple cider vinegar is and how lucky I am to have gotten to know it so well.

The benefits are numerous, and we have gone through quite a lot of them. Whether you are the sort of person who is always worried about excessive weight and those extra pounds making an appearance, or you are the kind of person who is merely looking for a fresher take on life, apple cider vinegar is your answer.

Yes, apple cider vinegar is no stranger to controversies and critics. Some continue to claim that it is nothing more than an acidic drink poised to destroy you from the inside out. It does cause a bit of concern when you look at the number of these people as they are in thousands.

This is yet another reason why I decided to pick this project up and address the naysayers once and for all; apple cider vinegar is nothing like they say it to be. Yes, an excess of anything is harmful. Even drinking too much water can lead to fatal consequences. I am not the person who would encourage anyone to use anything excessively as I fully understand how severe the outcomes can be.

With that said, though, when appropriately used, apple cider vinegar can boast a wide array of benefits. These include and are not limited to:

- It helps with stomach upsets
- Soothes a sore throat
- Lowers cholesterol
- Prevents indigestion
- Aids in weight loss
- Gets rid of dandruff
- Helps get rid of acne

- Boosts energy
- Helps control blood sugar levels

These are just at the tip of the iceberg, and there is much more to be explored. It should be of no surprise that the world continues to invest heavily in research to fully understand the benefits and any possible side effects of this incredible elixir that has been around for thousands of years.

Unlike some articles, blogs, and books I have come across, I wanted to remain as fair as possible by covering both aspects. As a consumer of ACV, you should know what goes into your body and if it is any good. I am happy to report that apple cider vinegar continues to defy the naysayers and prove just why it keeps sticking around.

It can be used on its own, although the taste might be a bit strong, or it can be used to create some refreshing drinks. If you are feeling a bit adventurous, use apple cider vinegar as a component for a recipe you may have read on the internet. You will be surprised at how well the apple cider vinegar brings the taste to life.

Typically, athletes and celebrities avoid opting for things that are marred by and riddled with controversies. For apple cider vinegar, the list of athletes and celebrities backing the drink continues to grow in number. With incredibly famous people, like Jennifer Aniston, using ACV to maintain their gorgeous looks and figure, it leaves no room for doubt. ACV is genuinely the find of a lifetime and does what it claims to do best.

Whether you aim to take the longer route of making your own home-made apple cider vinegar or buy one from the shelf, this will undoubtedly change the way you live. Combine it with some holistic living and a fitness routine, and the results will leave you and those around you staggered.

Whenever you aim to begin your journey into the world of ACV, I would recommend either buying a good quality apple cider vinegar with the mother or creating your own with the mother. Having that layer of gelatinous substance that floats around or settles down at the bottom of the bottle ensures that you get the maximum nutrition and benefits every time you use the apple cider vinegar.

Throughout the years, I have advised people to use ACV, and I have observed that two of the most common reasons why people use ACV have to do with either losing weight or bringing their blood sugar levels under control. Whichever reason you may have, I assure you that the results are well worth it.

The key to a successful journey lies not in the quantity of apple cider vinegar, but it is the consistency that matters the most. If you are looking for overnight results, it is best to turn away. Every good thing takes time to manifest itself. Perseverance, consistency, and determination are what will guarantee your success.

Mark your calendars down accordingly and take your measurements the day you start. Six months later, come back and prepare to scream in joy as you rediscover the better side of yourself. The person that once stood with a belly popping out and some misplaced pounds would now be a sharp, glowing, and attractive-looking person who you never thought you would ever see again.

For the people who may be suffering from diabetes or heart conditions, apple cider vinegar will do you wonders. However, before you decide to make a leap of faith, consider talking to a doctor as there are medications known to interact with apple cider vinegar. It is always best to be sure that your medicine would not interact and hence amplify any side effects.

As long as you are given the green light, apple cider vinegar will be your source of renewed energy, a more energized you, and a better immune system that's ready to fend off bacteria, ailments, and diseases.

Finally, for the people who may have been suffering from hair loss issues or acne-related problems, you can apply diluted apple cider vinegar topically to produce some of the most exciting results. Some celebrities vouch for the results, and that is saying something.

"Life is not merely being alive, but being well." - Marcus Valerius Martialis

Remember that apple cider vinegar alone cannot do much for you except keep some of your body's components in check. To truly experience the finest results, incorporate a healthy lifestyle, pick up some healthy exercise routines, and follow them religiously. Sooner than later, you will realize just how much you have been missing out on.

If you are reading this, I have every confidence to say that you have what it takes to step up and reclaim your healthy lifestyle. Do not let anyone tell you otherwise. The right path is often the one less walked upon, not because people don't know of it, but because people are told otherwise and led to believe that the path is wrong.

Yes, it will take time, but I assure you, with the kind of determination you showed while reading this book, you have all it takes to be the next success story. I love the idea of helping people out, and I love the idea of getting direct feedback from my readers about their success stories even more. I will eagerly be waiting to hear you say, "Yes, it worked!"

Till that time, I bid you farewell and hope that one day this book helps you regain what you thought was lost for good. Never give up; never look back. The only way is up and forward!

References

Appenbrink, K. (2016, April 20). 21 ways to cook with apple cider vinegar. Retrieved from https://www.thekitchn.com/20-recipes-that-make-use-of-apple-cider-vinegar-230195

Bubnis, D. (2020, February 26). The numbers behind obesity. Retrieved from https://www.medicalnewstoday.com/articles/319902#the-cost-of-obesity

Burry, M. (2018, August 13). 6 ways to use apple cider vinegar for more beautiful hair. Retrieved from https://www.prevention.com/beauty/hair/a22709576/apple-cider-vinegar-for-hair/

Butler, N. (2018, April 25). 6 essential nutrients and why your body needs them. Retrieved from https://www.healthline.com/health/food-nutrition/six-essential-nutrients

Christiano, D. (2018, June 20). Corticosteroids and Weight Gain: What You Need to Know. Retrieved from https://www.healthline.com/health/steroids-and-weight-gain

Diabetes Statistics. (n.d.). Retrieved from https://www.diabetesresearch.org/diabetes-statistics

Heart Disease Facts. (2019, December 2). Retrieved from https://www.cdc.gov/heartdisease/facts.htm

How a Healthy Heart Can Benefit Your Brain: Tri-City Medical Center. (2018, December 29). Retrieved from https://www.tricitymed.org/2017/10/healthy-heart-can-benefit-brain/

Marengo, K. (2018, November 16). Health benefits of apple cider vinegar. Retrieved from https://www.medicalnewstoday.com/articles/323721

Melero, A. (2019, June 24). I drank apple cider vinegar for a week every morning because Jennifer Aniston swears by it - Here's what happened. Retrieved from https://www.thezoereport.com/p/i-drank-apple-cider-vinegar-for-a-week-every-morning-because-jennifer-aniston-swears-by-it-heres-what-happened-18137178

Panoff, L. (2019, June 26). Is drinking apple cider vinegar before bed beneficial? Retrieved from https://www.healthline.com/nutrition/apple-cider-vinegar-before-bed

Quinn, J. (2020, January 19). I drank apple cider vinegar every day to lose weight and the results were shocking. Retrieved from https://www.cheatsheet.com/health-fitness/apple-cider-vinegar-weight-loss.html/

Samad, Anuar & Azlan, Azrina & A, Ismail. (2016). Therapeutic Effects of Vinegar: A Review. Current Opinion in Food Science. 8. 10.1016/j.cofs.2016.03.001.

Made in United States
Cleveland, OH
04 November 2026

47642859R00087